Exercises in Radiological Diagnosis

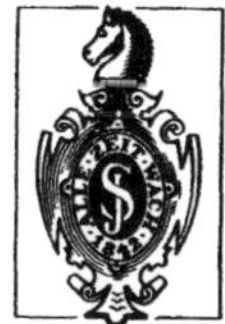

J.-F. Bonneville F. Cattin

Cervical Spine: Tricks and Traps

60 Radiological Exercises for Students and Practitioners

With 199 Illustrations

Springer-Verlag Berlin Heidelberg New York
London Paris Tokyo Hong Kong

Prof. Dr. Jean-Francois Bonneville
Dr. Francoise Cattin
Département de Neuroradiologie et de Radiologie Ostéo-Articulaire
Centre Hospitalier Universitaire de Besançon
Hôpital Jean Minjoz
Boulevard Fleming
F-25030 Besançon

Illustrations by Michel Gaudron

ISBN-13:978-3-540-17683-1 e-ISBN-13:978-3-642-72584-5
DOI: 10.1007/978-3-642-72584-5

Library of Congress Cataloging-in-Publication Data. Bonneville, Jean-François, 1943– Cervical spine: tricks and traps : 60 radiological exercises for students and practitioners / J.-F. Bonneville, F. Cattin. p. cm.–(Exercises in radiological diagnosis) Translated from the French.
ISBN-13:978-3-540-17683-1
1. Vertebrae, Cervical–Radiography–Problems, exercises, etc. 2. Spine–Radiography–Problems, exercises, etc. 3. Vertebrae, Cervical–Tomography–Problems, exercises, etc. 4. Spine–Tomography–Problems, exercises, etc. I. Cattin, F. II. Title. III. Series. [DNLM: 1. Cervical Vertebrae–radiography–problems. WE 18 B717c] RD531.B66 1990 616.3'750757–dc20 DNLM/DLC 90-9462 CIP

2127/3130-543210 – Printed on acid-free paper

Preface

The cervical spine is always examined initially using standard radiographs, which often provide a sufficient basis for diagnosis.

Malformations, tumours, more frequently trauma, rheumatism, and even plain neck pain require a radiological examination.

The interpretation of radiological images is often difficult because of overlapping pieces of bone, the summation phenomena and the diversity of projections.

In this book, two- or three-dimensional CT scans accompany the standard radiographs, serving as an excellent aid for comprehension. It is almost as if the reader actually had the bones shown in the radiographs in his hands.

From then on, everything becomes easy, superimpositions vanish, traps come to light, anatomy triumphs, and the images takes on life.

Besançon, 1990 J.-F. Bonneville, F. Cattin

Contents

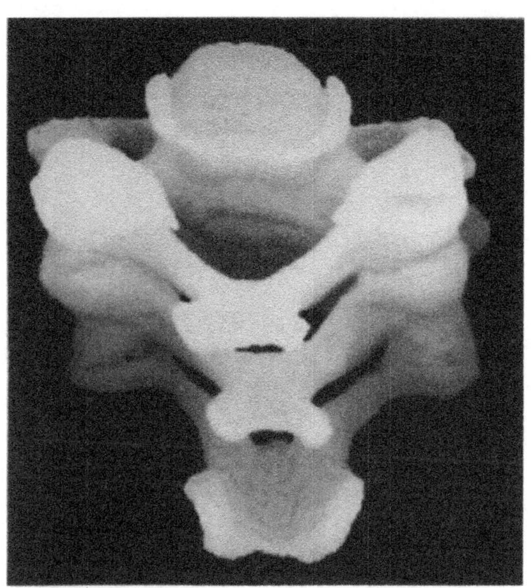

Normal cervical spine:
3-D imaging

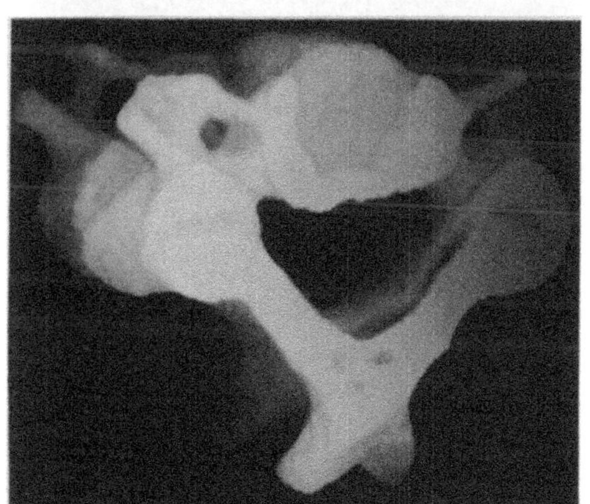

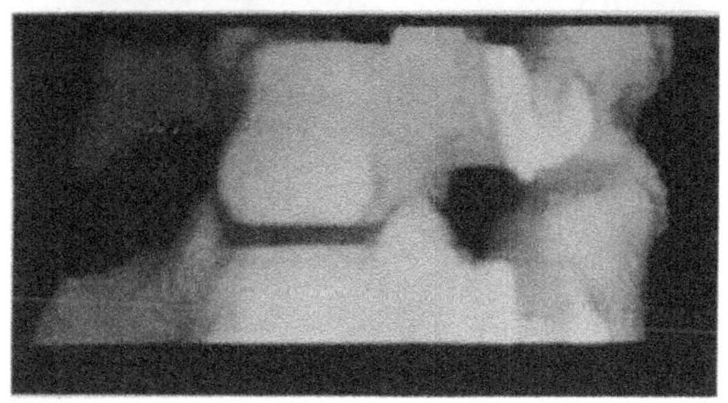

1

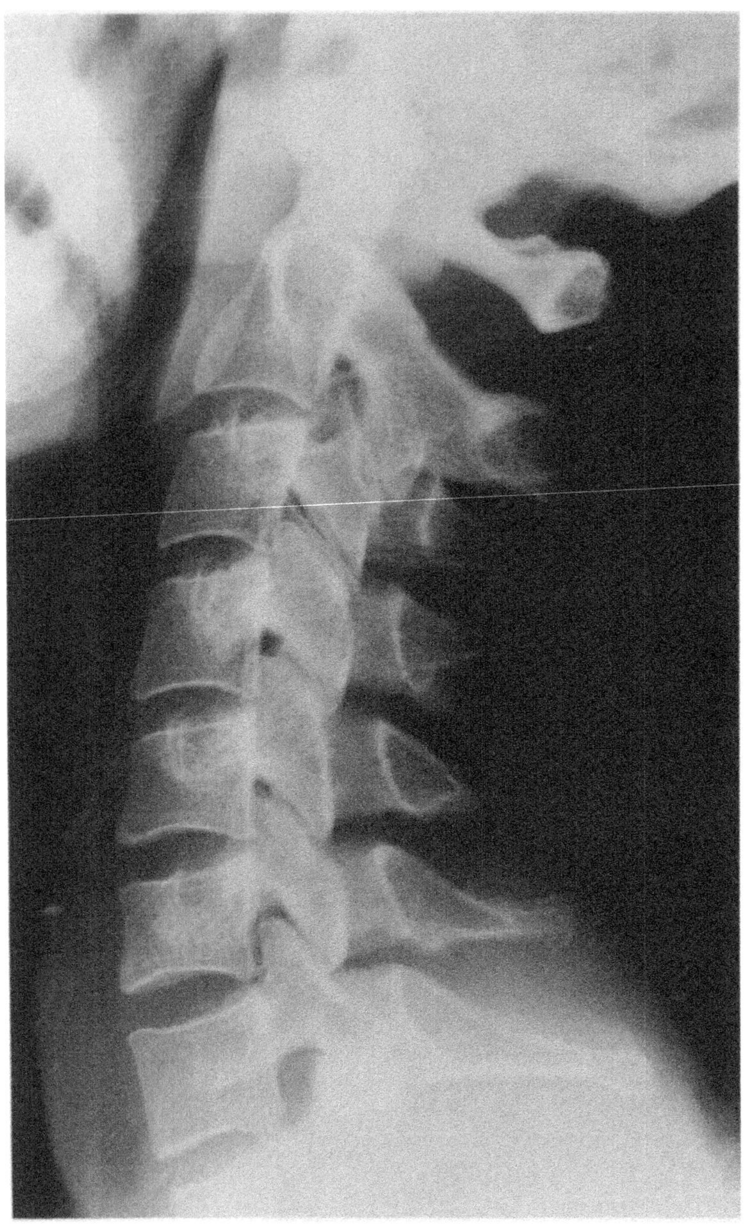

Our starting point is a normal lateral radiograph of the cervical spine. It will serve as a guide and point of reference in our task of comprehending the interrelationships between the structures of the cervical spine. This radiograph correctly includes the entire area from the base of the skull to the cervicothoracic junction. The soft tissues are clearly visible anteriorly, as are the extremities of the spinous processes posteriorly. In this case, with the subject looking straight ahead, is a slight, regular, physiological lordosis of the cervical column.

Let us now list the important points which should be automatically analysed on a lateral radiograph of the cervical spine. Modifications in the prevertebral soft tissues constitute a valuable sign in cases of cervical trauma. These modifications are rarely absent in lesions of the anterior part of the vertebral bodies, the discs, or the anterior longitudinal ligament. Under normal technical conditions, the thickness of the prevertebral soft tissue is less than 4 to 5 mm at the anteroinferior angles of C2 and C3; a thickness of 7 mm is very suspicious. Caudal to C4 and C5, the retrotracheal space is very much larger owing to the interposition of the oesophagus; a thickness of up to 17 mm is not suspicious.

Two major complementary relationships are of practical interest. The posterior wall of the nasopharynx is always concave or flat at the level of C2. At the level of the base of the odontoid process, the prevertebral soft tissues are almost always less than or equal to the anteroposterior diameter of the odontoid process.

The anterior and posterior surfaces of the vertebral bodies form one continous line, as does the spinolaminar line situated at the junction of the laminae on the midline. At each stage, the spinolaminar line is neatly formed and often forms a discrete posterior concavity. On lateral views, the transverse process is projected onto the vertebral bodies: from C3 to C6, the projection of the anterior tubercle of the transverse process is seen as a thin, dense, vertical line superimposed on the superior half of the vertebral body and the adjacent disc. Most often, the right and left anterior tubercles can be seen separately. In comparison, the vertebral body of C7 appears bare as there are no anterior tubercles on the transverse processes.

The intervertebral foramina are not visible in the lateral view, except at C2–C3 and, most often, at C7–T1. At C7–T1, the intervertebral foramen is partially visible in the lateral view as the superior articular process of T1 is situated more anteriorly than that of the cervical vertebrae owing to the different morphology and orientation of the pedicles of T1. Anywhere else, the diamond-shaped articular processes normally project up to the plane of the posterior surfaces of the vertebral bodies and fill the foramen, resulting in the nonvisualisation of the intervertebral foramen.

The space between the posterior surface of the articular process and the spinolaminar line is called "the safety space"; it is normally always present and measures 5 mm on average. Appreciation of this safety space is essential for the diagnosis of stenosis and enlargement of the cervical spinal canal. The pedicles are not normally visible in the lateral view at the cervical level. All of these features will be dealt with in detail in the following exercises.

2

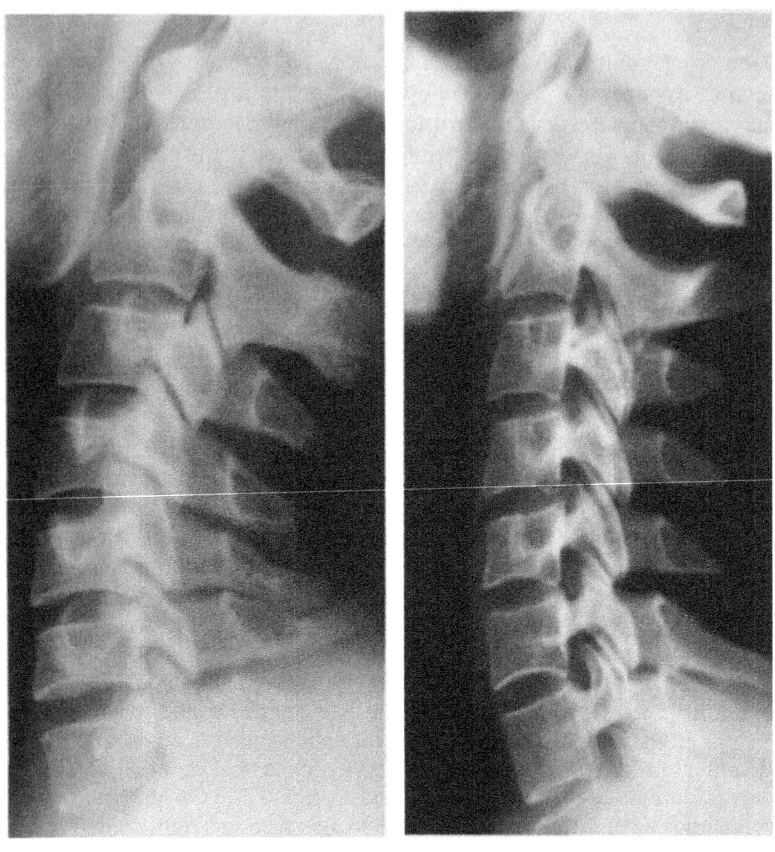

a b

These two radiographs of the cervical spine present some anatomical variations. Analyse each of the relationships described in case 1.

a The articular processes of C4, C5 and C6 largely overlap the vertebral bodies and the adjacent discs. This anterior position of the articular processes is the result of a particular anatomical variation of the pedicles which are shorter and are orientated almost transversally. **c** It is possible to see that this anatomical variation is responsible for the narrow appearance of the intervertebral foramen. Compare this with the normal appearance (**d**).

b On the other hand, the pedicles of the vertebrae C3–C7 have an anteroposterior orientation and are thus visible on a lateral radiograph. This results in the articular processes being located more posteriorly than usual and in partial visualisation of the intervertebral foramina (**d**). If you have carefully studied all the relationships, you will have also discovered another anatomical variation: in this case, the anterior tubercle of the transverse process of C6 is missing.

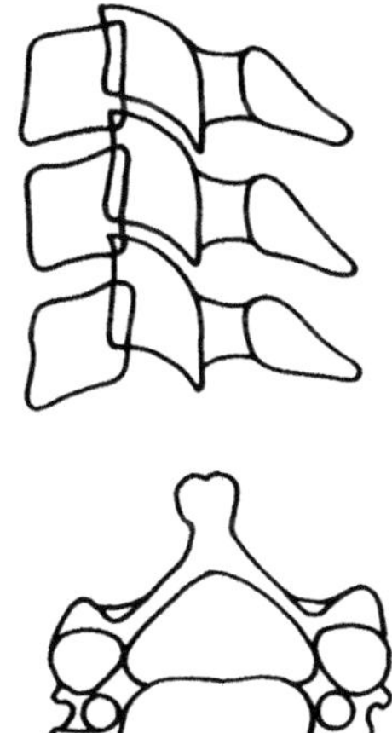

c

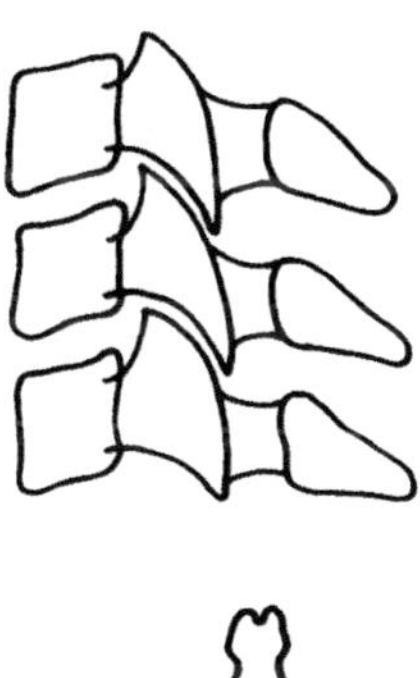

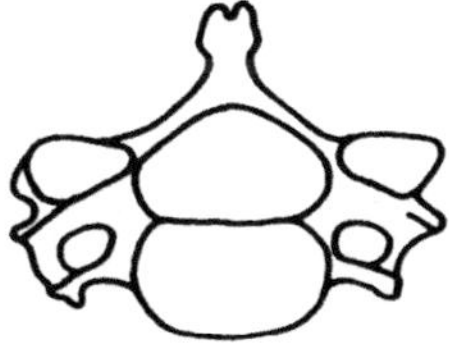

d

3

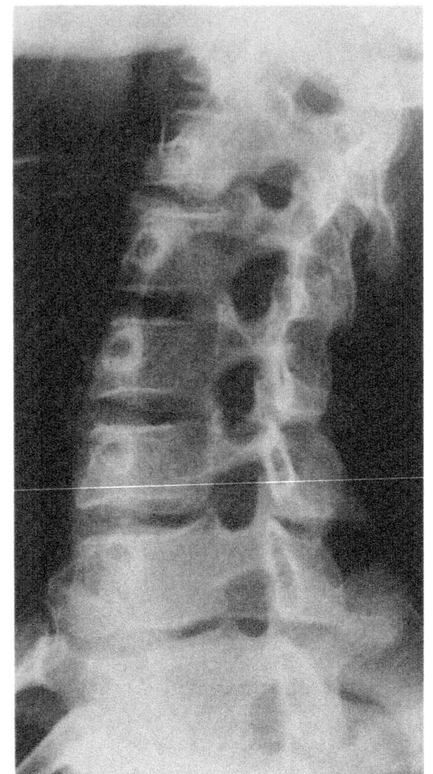

a

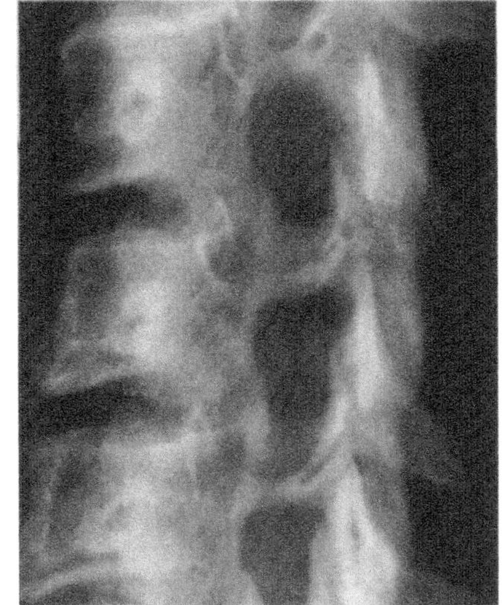

b

Here is an oblique view of the cervical spine (**a**). This projection enables the visualisation of the intervertebral foramina; we shall return to this in just a moment. First of all, train yourself to make sure that the pedicles opposite the intervertebral foramina are present and correctly aligned, for example, in this case the pedicles on the right. It is at this projection that the "eye" of the vertebra should be looked for.

The left intervertebral foramina shown here are clearly bounded superiorly and inferiorly by the pedicles of the adjacent vertebrae. Thus, the size of the intervertebral foramen depends on the morphology of the pedicles: if the pedicles are small and thick, the foramina are small. On the other hand, if the pedicles are long and thin, the foramina are large.

b You will have already recognised the constitutionally large intervertebral foramina because the pedicles are long and thin at several levels as well as bilaterally. Note that the right pedicles appear also small in configuration.

You are now familiar with the essential anatomical relationships as seen on lateral and oblique views of the cervical spine. Do not hesitate to refer frequently to these first pages throughout your reading. From now on, carefully look at the figures which are on the left page. Answer the questions at the top of the page on the right while covering the answers with a piece of paper.

Good luck!

4

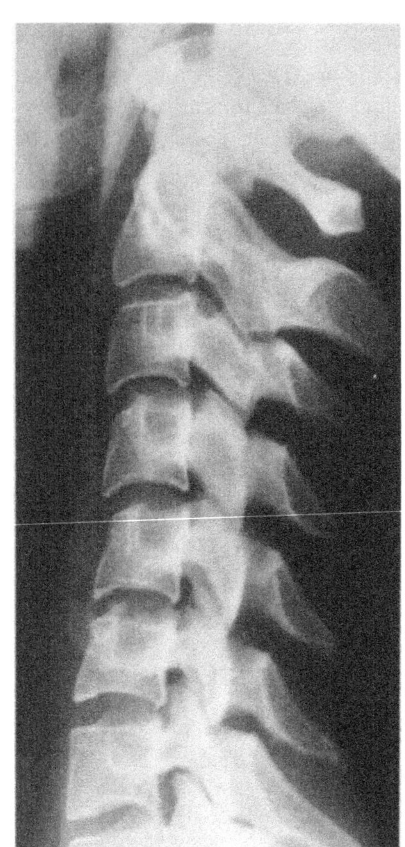

a

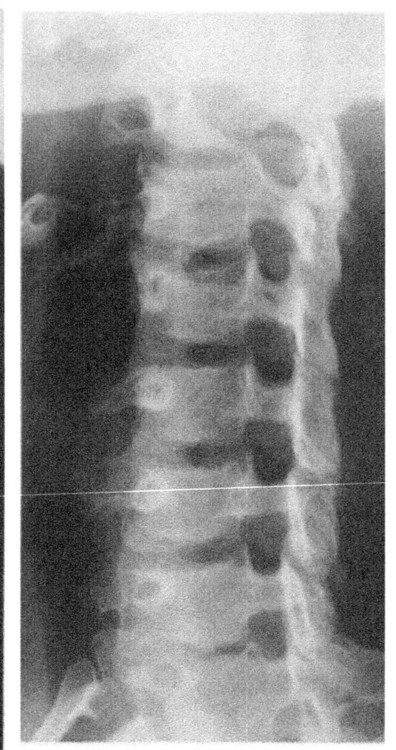

b

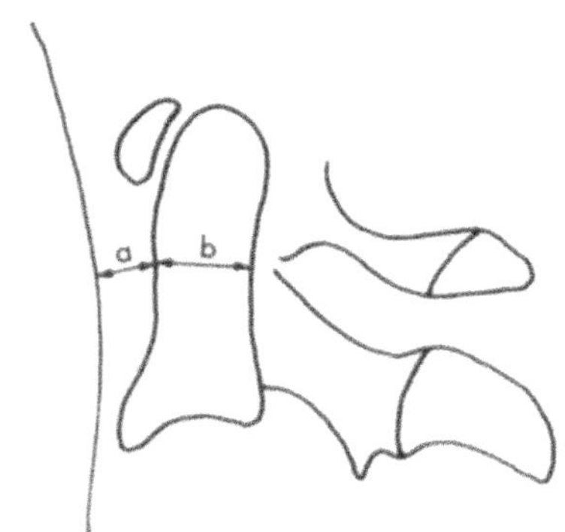

c

Here is a final piece of revision before starting. **a, b** These lateral and oblique views of the same patient are almost normal. Look carefully at all the essential features: the soft tissues, the anterior and posterior surfaces of the vertebrae, the position of the articular processes, the safety space, the spinolaminar line, the intervertebral foramina and both pedicles. You should notice two features here because they are different from the previous descriptions.

First, the cervical lordosis is not present: this is common in a normal subject who stiffens a little during the X-.ray exposure. Secondly, there is an osseous image in front of the anterior aspect of the body of C6, corresponding to a slight hypertrophy of the transverse process which is well visualised in the lateral and the oblique views. You will have certainly noted that the body of C7 is bare because there is no anterior tubercle of the transverse process on this vertebra. Note also that the body of C7 is frequently larger and more square-shaped than that of the vertebrae above. Let us use these last normal radiographs to formulate some complementary relationships:

- The anterior arch of atlas is in contact with the anterior surface of the odontoid process.
- The spinolaminar line of C2 is normally situated 1 or 2 mm posterior to those of the neighbouring vertebrae.

And now an important reminder which we shall require shortly: the thickness of the soft tissues in front of C2 is less than, or equal to the anteroposterior diameter of the base of the odontoid process (**c**).

5

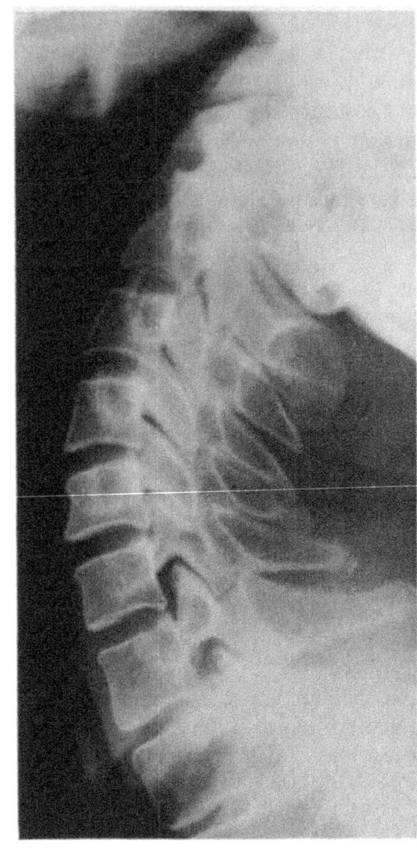

a

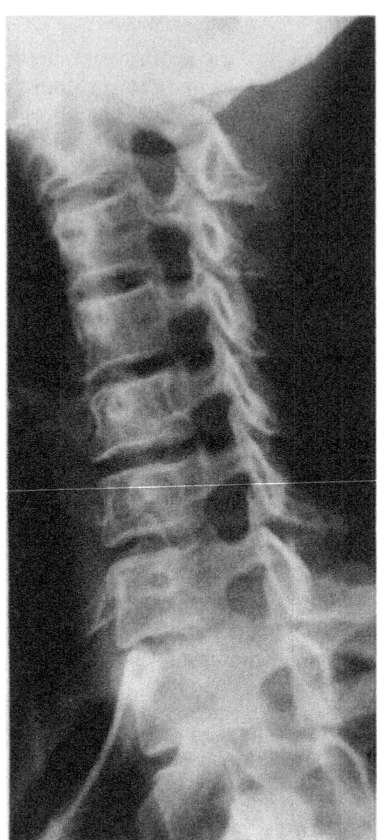

b

Have you remembered everything? Good! We can now begin. From now on, do not forget to cover the part of the page situated below the line. The hyperlordosis of the cervical spine is not significant: the lateral view was taken with extension of the head. What do you notice here?

The feature that should have drawn your attention here is that the intervertebral foramen of C6–C7 is partially visible in the lateral view (**a**), which is unusual. The explanation is that we are looking at a transitional anomaly of the cervicothoracic junction. C7 is transformed, presenting the characteristics of thoracic vertebrae: the body of C7 is large and square, and the orientation of the pedicles is similar to those in the thoracic region. As a result, the superior articular processes are situated more posteriorly than usual, thus making the C6–C7 intervertebral foramen partially visible.

The "thoracisation" of C7 is confirmed in the oblique projection where we can see a small cervical rib (**b**). In this case, C6 slightly resembles the usual appearance of the C7 vertebra; the body of C6 is square, and there is no anterior tubercle of the transverse process. It should be reemphasised that it is the intervertebral foramen of C7–T1 which is usually visible on the lateral view. In the case of a transitional anomaly of the cervicothoracic region, the intervertebral foramen at C6–C7 may become partially visible on the lateral view.

6

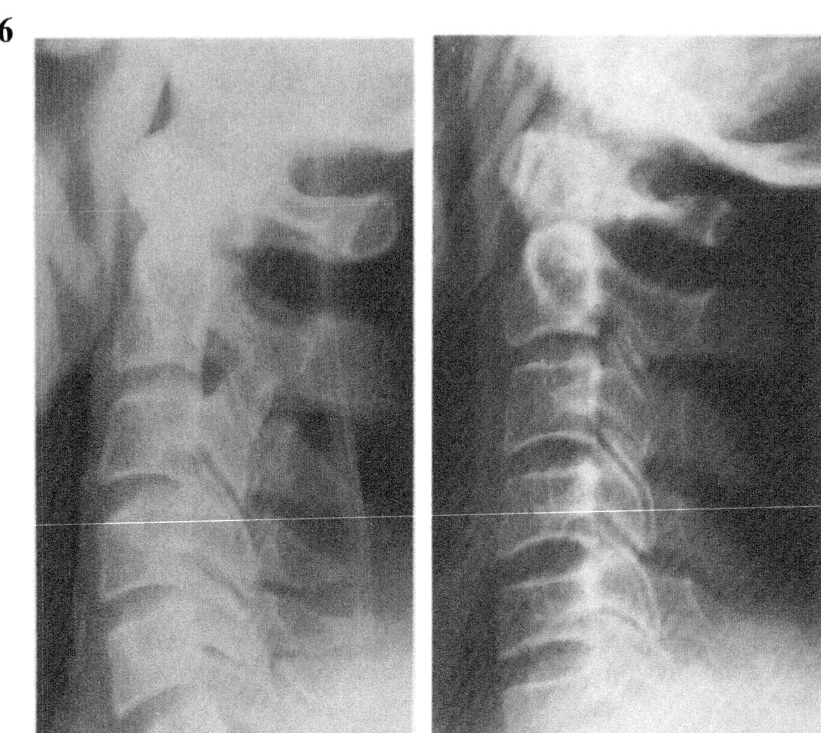

Case 6

Here are the radiographs (**a, b**) of two patients who were admitted to hospital in a coma following a traffic accident. You are asked to determine whether vertebral trauma, possibly associated with head injury, has occurred.

As is possible in an emergency, the radiographs are not technically perfect. In these circumstances the methods of interpretation discussed earlier should be used.

A systematic study of the two radiographs will have allowed you to see that the vertebral bodies are properly aligned. This immediately enables you to verify the normality of the prevertebral soft tissues, in particular at C2, which practically eliminates the possibility of a fracture of the odontoid process. In the case of multiple injuries, a search for a lesion at the cervicothoracic junction, which, as here, is often hidden by the shoulders, should be a priority for the radiologist. You should have therefore already realised that in these two cases the intervertebral foramen at C6–C7 is empty, signifying that the articular process of C7 is not in its place, and, in fact, if you look carefully, you will find it in each case behind the inferior articular process of C6, thus abnormally occupying the safety space.

In each case, a second radiograph obtained with the shoulders pulled down (or a tomogram or CT scan) confirmed the fracture-dislocation (**c**).

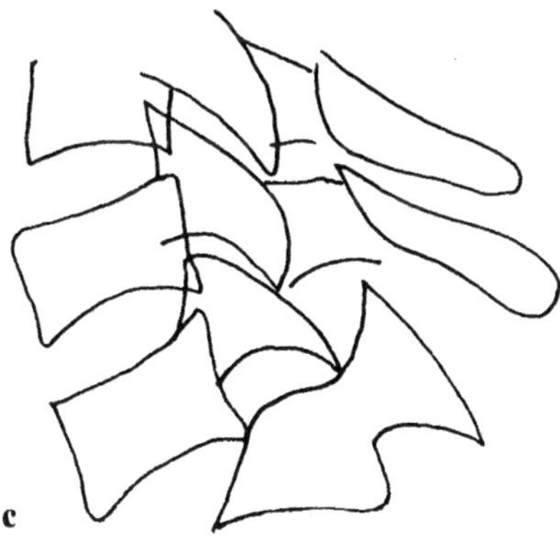

c

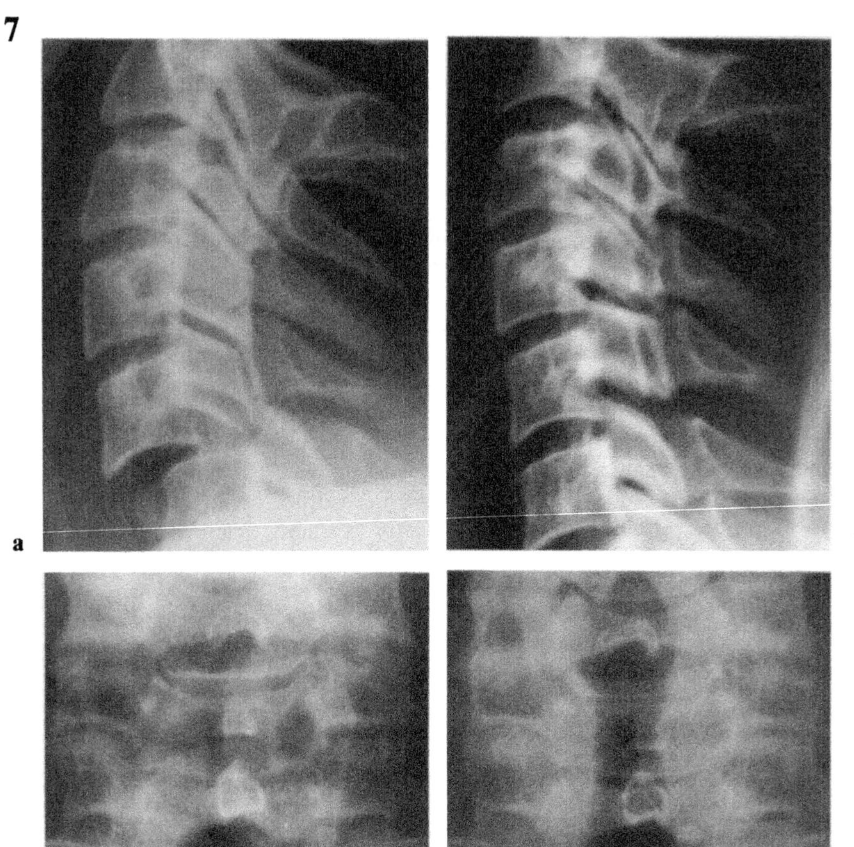

The diagnosis of dislocation with locking of the articular processes is generally much easier at C5–C6 than at C6–C7 or C7–T1 because of the projection of the shoulders. Radiograph **b** was obtained a few hours after **a**, after reduction by orthopaedic treatment. What are the abnormal radiological signs in **b**? Also, which is the initial frontal projection, **c** or **d**?

In **b** we note an abnormal increase in the articular joint space at C5–C6 and also at C4–C5, indicating that the articular capsule has been strained. There is also an abnormal opening in the interlaminar space of C5–C6, indicating a tear of the ligamenta flava, and in the interspinous space of C5–C6, indicating a tear in the interspinous ligament. **d** is the initial film as the interspinous distance of C6–C7 is greater here than in **c** (**e**). A vertebral dislocation with locking of the articular processes could be suspected in the frontal projection in view of the abnormal interspinous distance. However, an isolated fracture of the spinous process may produce a similar displacement (**f**).

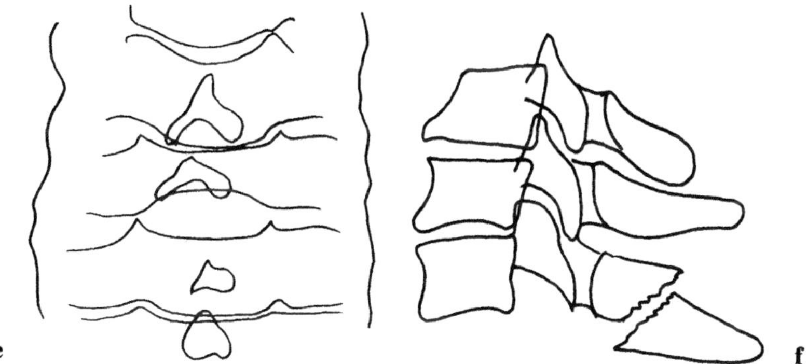

e f

8

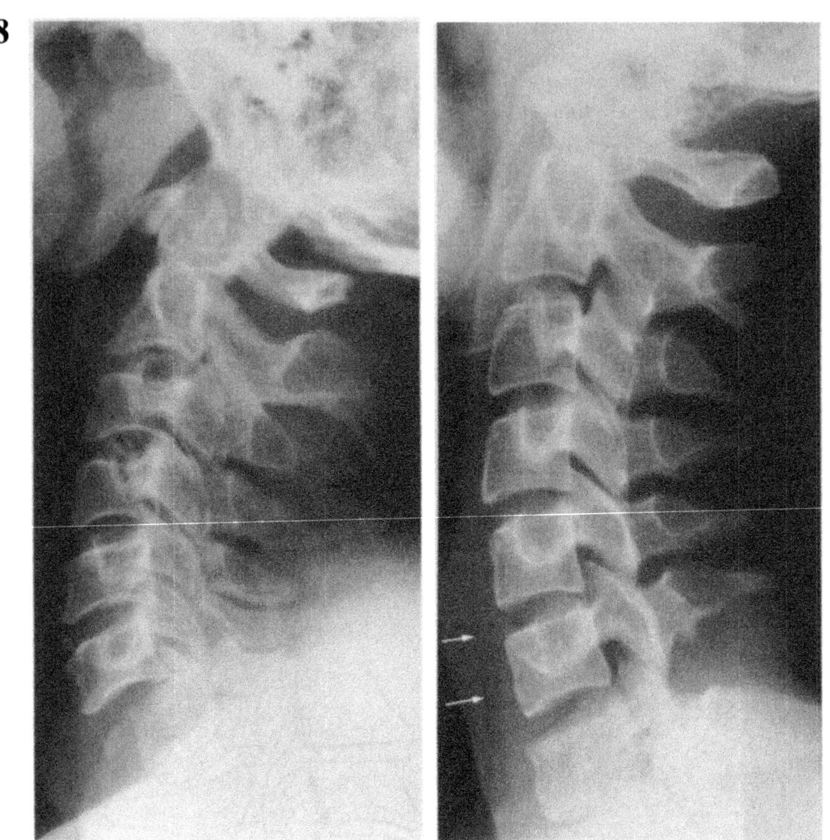

a b

Be careful! A superior articular process which is apparently correctly placed with respect to the intervertebral foramen at C6–C7 does not eliminate a severe injury at the cervicothoracic junction. Note carefully all the lesions which can be seen in **a** and **b**.

Always look carefully at the prevertebral soft tissues which are almost modified in the case of severe injury involving the anterior part of the cervical spine. **a** There is a clear increase in the thickness of the soft tissues in front of C6, indicating diffuse haemorrhage or oedema up to the level of C2. This thickening of the soft tissues may appear up to 24–48 h after the injury. It is difficult to appreciate this sign in the case of endotracheal intubation or if the film has been taken in deep inspiration or during swallowing. The body of C7 is displaced posteriorly, as is one of the articular processes which is projected onto the safety space. The other superior articular process is fractured at its base, but has remained in its normal position in front of the inferior articular process of C6. However, there is a pathological increase in the articular joint space at C6–C7, indicating a rupture of the articular capsule.

b The pharynx and the trachea are in place, but there is an anterior displacement of the radiolucent prevertebral fat line, situated in contact with the anterior surface of the longus colli, normally 1–2 mm in front of the anterior surface of the vertebral bodies *(arrows)*. The superior end-plate of C7 is compressed and there is an avulsion fracture of the inferior surface of the laminae of C6; the interlaminar space is enlarged, indicating a tear of the ligamenta flava, and an increase of size in the interspinous space, indicating a tear of the interspinous ligament. It is necessary to verify, by careful flexion and extension, the integrity of the C6–C7 articular capsules, and, by a tomogram or a CT scan, the integrity of the superior articular processes of C7.

9

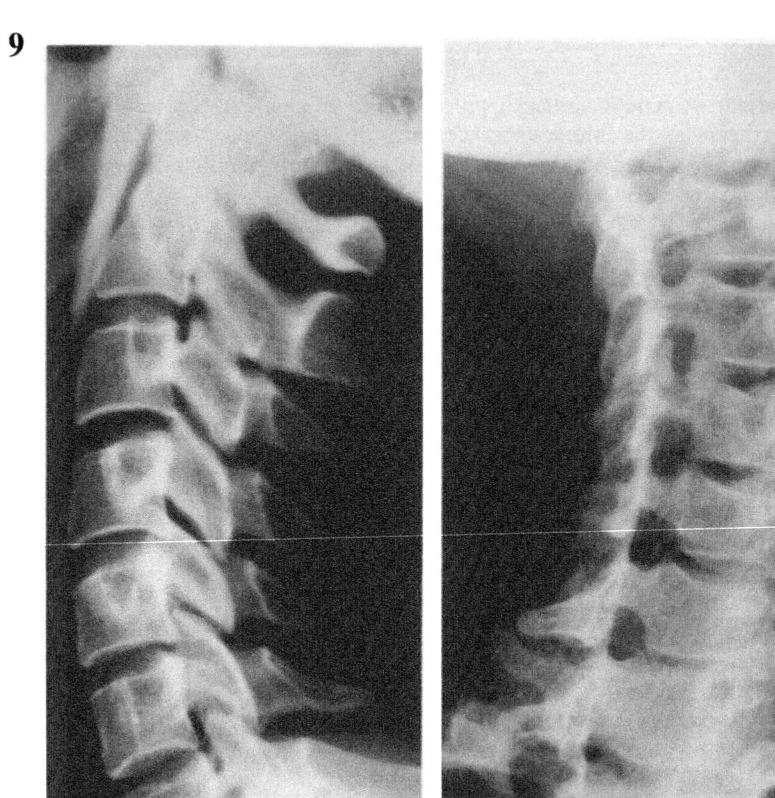

a b

One of the intervertebral foramina, visualised here in the oblique view (**b**), is clearly smaller than the others. Which one? Why? Which is the nerve root which is possibly under threat in this intervertebral foramen?

The right C4–C5 intervertebral foramen is small. The C5 root passes through this foramen (remember that the C8 root passes through the C7–T1 foramen). The reason for this narrow intervertebral foramen is revealed in the lateral view (**a**) where we can clearly see that the superior articular process of C5 is located much further forward than the others. Note again, in the three-dimensional CT scan (**c**), the anterior position of the superior articular process resulting in the narrowed intervertebral foramen. Compare this with the usual pattern, for example, in page 1.

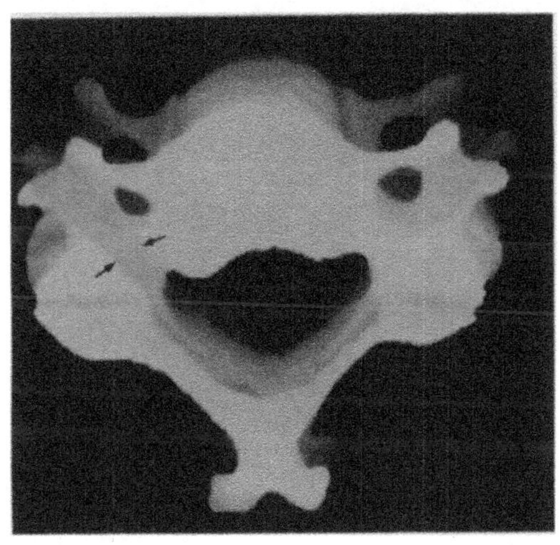

c

10

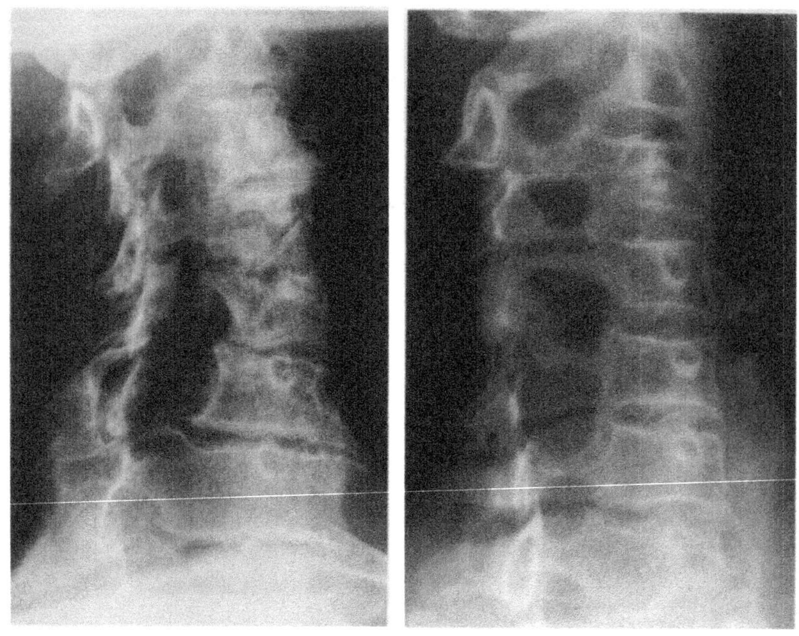

a

Here are abnormal intervertebral foramina in two patients. What do they make you think of?

First of all, you should have thought of a cervical neuroma, in which case you would be correct, at least in **a**: the C5–C6 and C6–C7 foramina on the right are very much enlarged. The right C6 pedicle has totally disappeared; the right C5 pedicle is very much demineralised. The enlargement of the foramina is symmetric: the neuroma has caused a well-defined erosion of the posterolateral part of the vertebral body and of the articular process. These tumoral imprints are not demineralised.

b The C4–C5 and C5–C6 foramina are very much enlarged. The pedicle of C6 is displaced caudally and reduced in size; the C5 pedicle is reduced in size superiorly and inferiorly. The causative lesion is therefore not a single one but a double one, due to the origin of the lesion within *each* intervertebral foramen. Note that the vertebral bodies are actually hardly modified. A diagnosis of multiple neuromas could have been possible. However, the true diagnosis was meningocele, that is, a dilatation of the arachnoid sheath which accompanies the cervical nerve roots; this was proved by the enhanced CT scan (**c**). The diagnosis of cervical meningoceles must be considered in the presence of enlarged intervertebral foramina with scalloping of the superior and inferior aspects of the pedicles, sometimes bilaterally. However, other diagnoses still have to be eliminated, as we shall soon see.

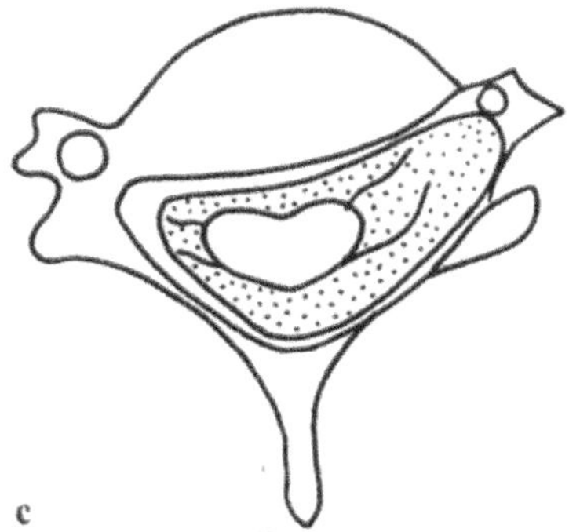

c

11

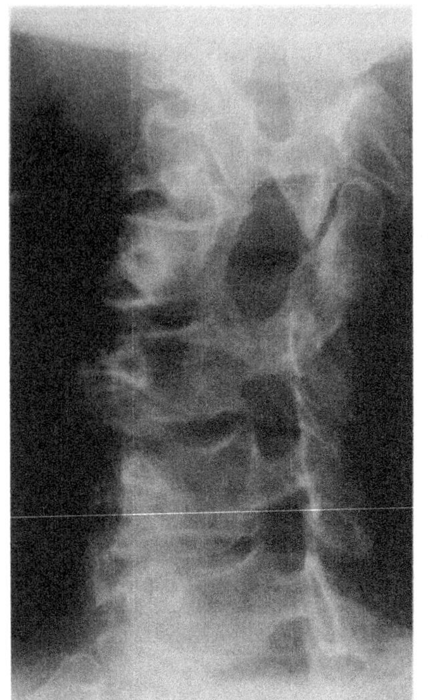

a

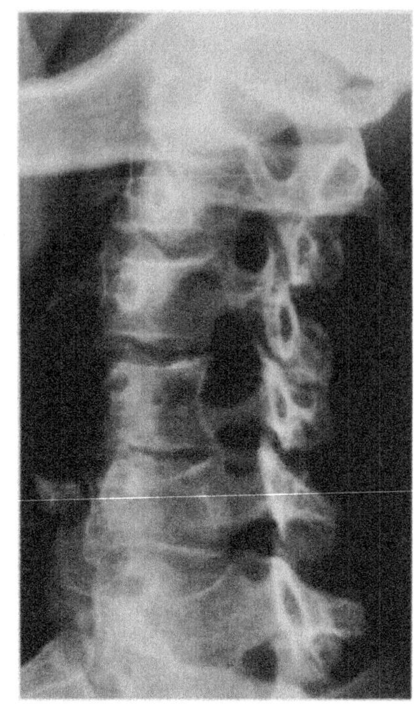

Here again there are two enlarged intervertebral foramina. To assist you: the patient in **b** presented with von Recklinghausen's neurofibromatosis.

---

a The left C4 pedicle is missing, but there is no sign of the adjacent osseous structures being compressed. The vertebral body is normal, as well is the pedicle below. On the other hand, we note a supplementary osseous structure which seems to articulate posteriorly with the inferior articular process of C3. It is a case of a complex vertebral malformation where the pedicle of C4 is missing, and the corresponding articular mass is displaced posteriorly. As can be seen in the three-dimensional CT scan (**c**), the lamina is orientated frontally *(arrow)*.

b The left C4–C5 foramen is enlarged; the left C5 pedicle is displaced caudally and thinned and there is a large imprint on the posterior part of the vertebral body. The contralateral pedicles are normal. The diagnosis of neurinoma could be suggested in the context of von Recklinghausen's disease, but we also have to think of an arteriovenous malformation at the expense of the vertebral artery, as in the case here. Therefore, when faced with von Recklinghausen's disease, we advices a systematic auscultation of the neck if an intervertebral foramen is found to be modified.

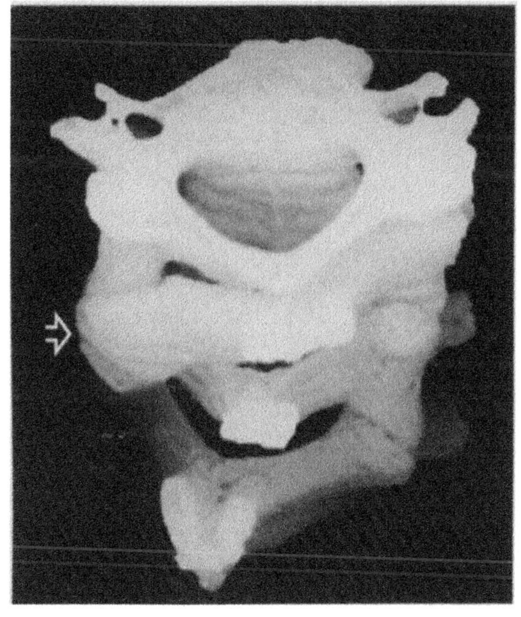

12

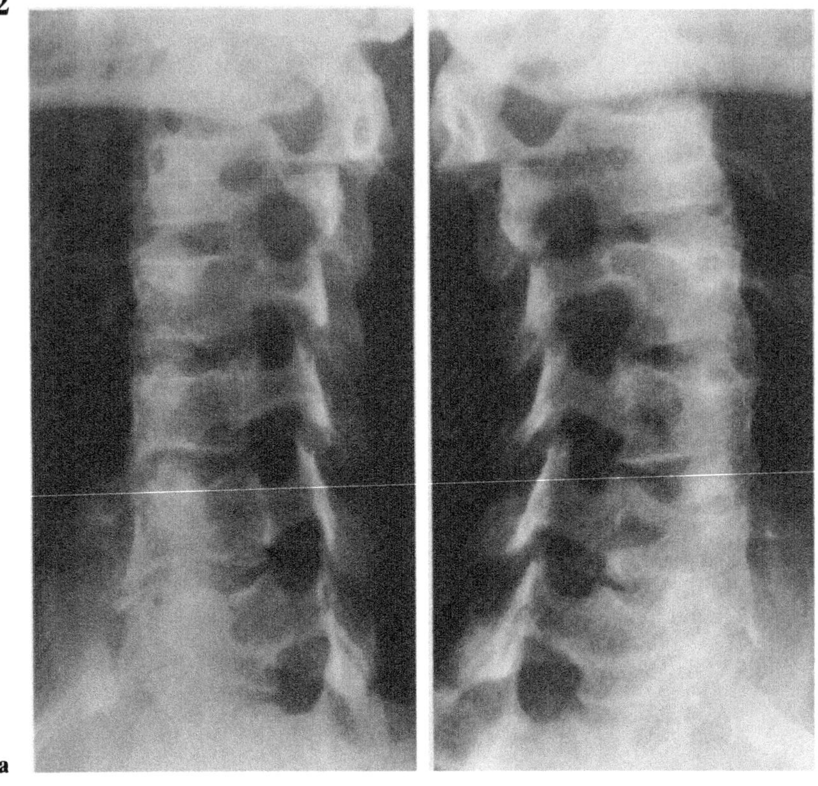

a

Case 12

The right C4–C5 intervertebral foramen is modiefied. What is the most likely diagnosis?

The right C4–C5 foramen is enlarged in its superior part (**b**) at the expense of the adjacent part of the vertebral body and the inferior aspect of the anterior part of the pedicle. The imprint on the vertebral body is rounded, very regular and finely encircled. All these features favour an image caused by a dolichovertebral artery, i.e. a nonpathological tortuosity of the vertebral artery. The presence of normal uncinate processes is also in favour of this diagnosis.

A diagnosis of neurinoma is very unlikely as the modifications are situated in the superior part of the intervertebral foramina, whereas the cervical nerve root is located immediately above the pedicle, namely the inferior part of the intervertebral foramen. Finally, the right C4 pedicle, which is well visualised "de face" in **a**, has been deformed into a crescent shape while its superior convexity has been preserved; these details are characteristic of a deformation associated with a dolichovertebral artery (**c**). The enhanced CT scan (**d**) confirms the diagnosis and explains the osseous deformations.

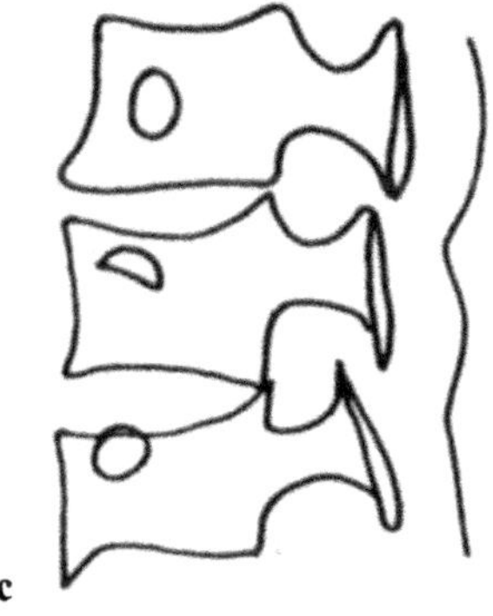

c

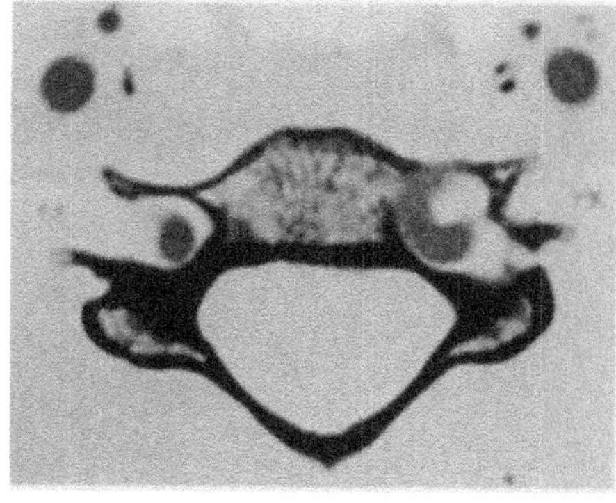

d

13

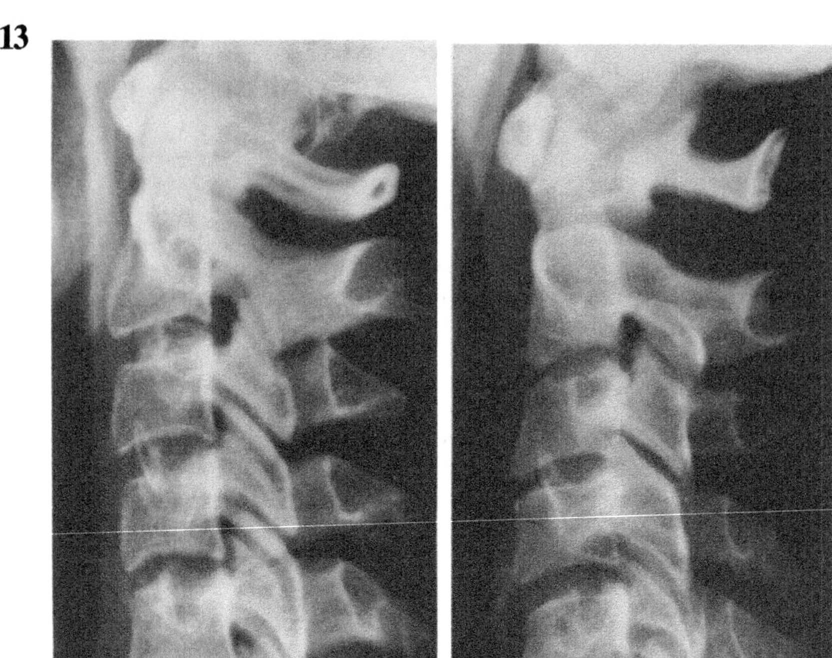

a

Case 13

Let us forget the intervertebral foramina for a moment. These two lateral radiographs of the cervical spine show the same anatomical variant. What is it?

You will have verified the alignment of the anterior and posterior margins of the vertebral bodies and the spinolaminar line, and you will have checked for the presence of the safety space, situated between the posterior surface of the articular process and the spinolaminar line. You will have certainly not forgotten the prevertebral soft tissues. You will have probably noticed that the spinous process of C3, C4 and C5 are much smaller than the others, as is frequently the case. And, if you have looked at the vertebral bodies themselves and the projection of the transverse processes, you will have certainly realised that in **a** and **b** C4 presents a horn-shaped osseous outgrowth corresponding to hypertrophy of the anterior tubercle of the transverse process which is perfectly demonstrated in the three-dimensional CT scans (**c–e**). It is a minor anatomical variant.

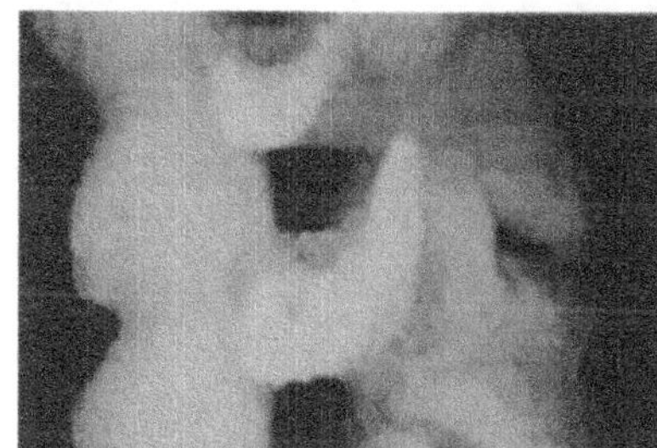

c

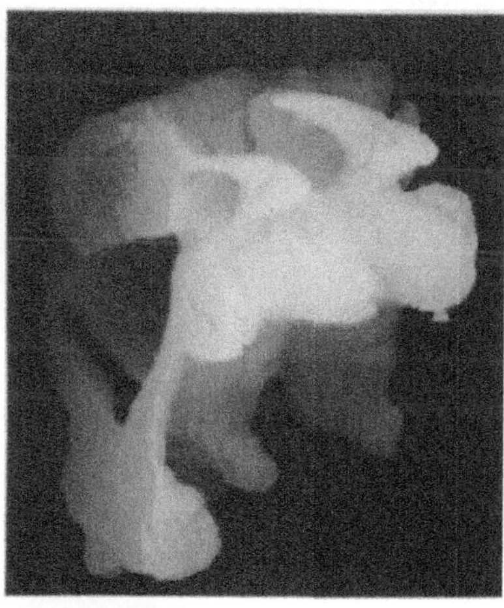

d

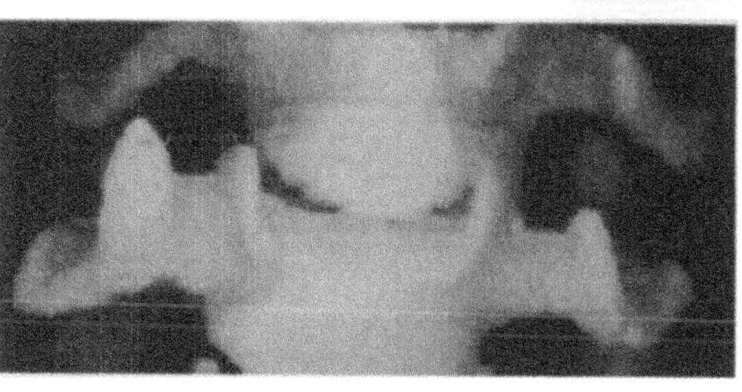

e

14

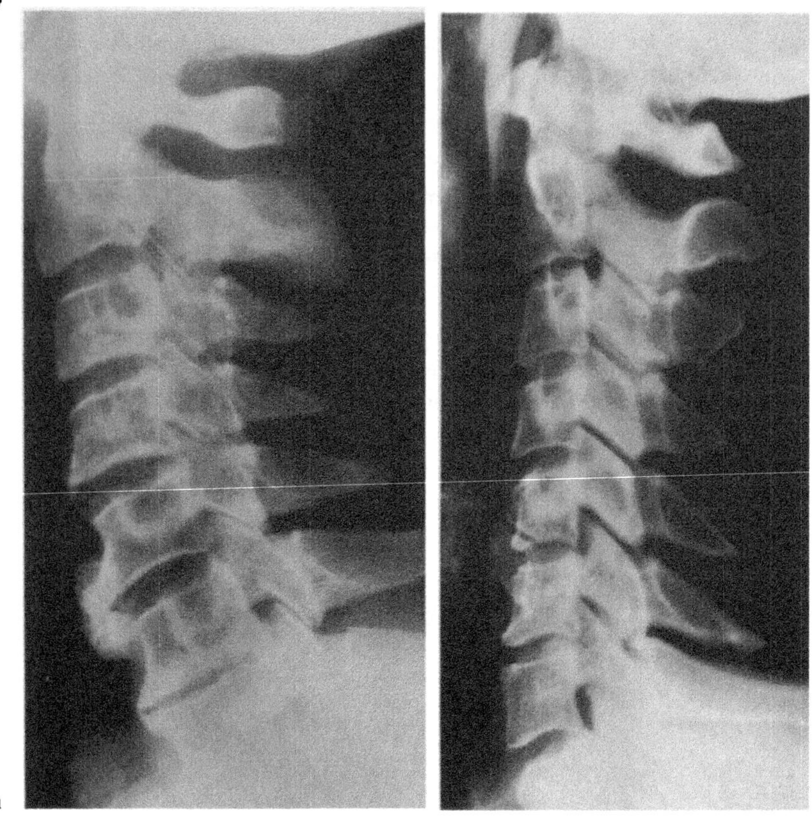

What is the difference between these two radiographs?

In fact, it should have been the similarity rather than the difference which caught your attention. In **a** as well as in **b**, you can see an abnormal osseous formation bridging C5 and C6 anteriorly. However, these formations are very different. In **a**, it is a case of giant osteophytes which are completely independent of the transverse processes as, in the lateral view, the projection of the normal anterior tubercles of these vertebrae can be seen very well. On the other hand, in **b**, it is not an osteophyte but a malformation: the transverse processes of C5 and C6 are hypertrophied and present an anterior neoarticulation, as demonstrated in the three-dimensional scan (**c**).

In fact, there are also other differences between the two radiographs, which you would have been able to spot if your analysis had been systematic. In **a**, the spinolaminar line of C2 is missing, as arch is not fused. On the other hand, there are alternating areas of sclerosis and osteolysis, indicating mixed metastatic lesions. Finally, the safety space is missing, particularly at C3, C4 and C5, indicating associated stenosis of the canal, which will be discussed later.

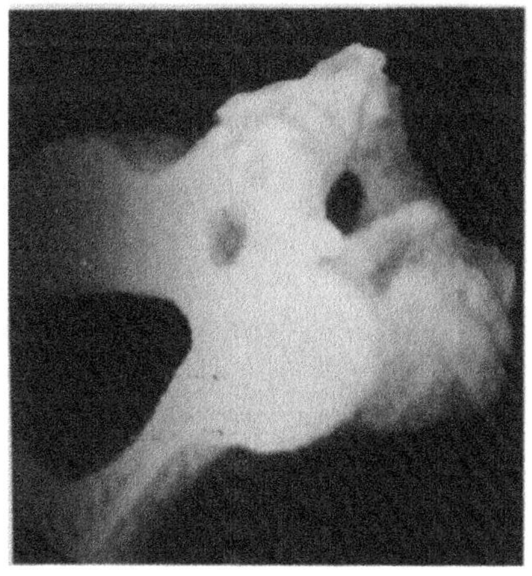

15

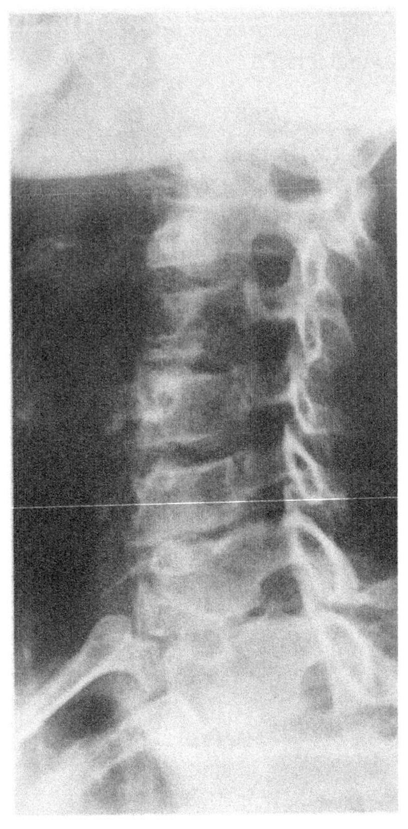

a

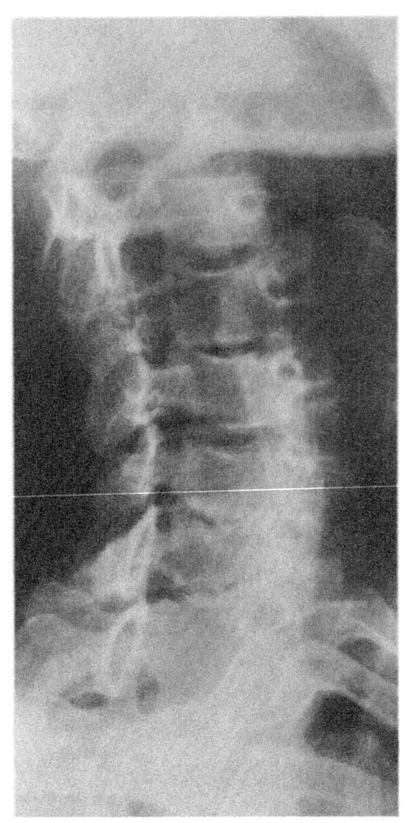

Let us return to the oblique radiographs: we know very well that these projections permit the visualisation of the intervertebral foramina, but we have already said that it is definitely more useful to examine first of all the ...

The pedicles! Had you remembered this, you would have noted that the right C4 pedicle is demineralised and that this abnormality is more evident when the pedicle is viewed "de face" (**a**) than when it is viewed from the side (**b**). This is a case of osteolytic metastasis from breast carcinoma; metastasis to the pedicle is often a first step. The osteolysis is perfectly demonstrated on the three-dimensional CT scan (**c**). In looking for metastasis to the cervical spine, bone scintigraphy is often less useful as degenerative changes may also give rise to "hot spots".

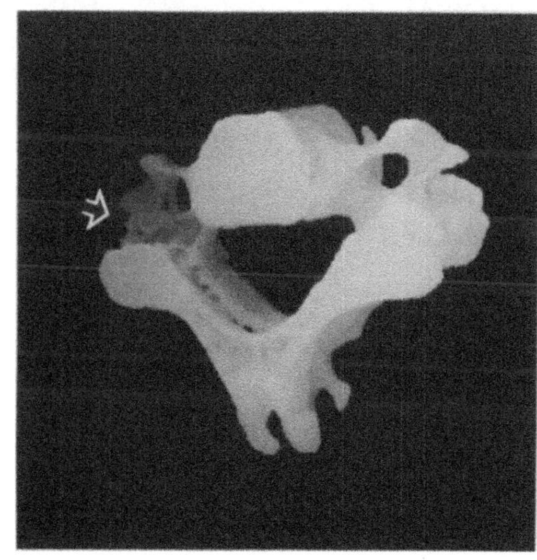

c

16

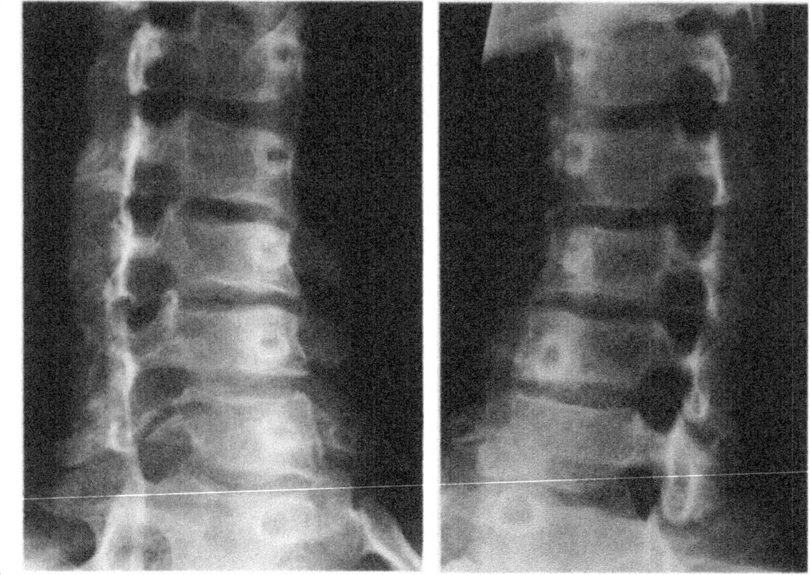

a

And here?

You will have again noted that there is a pedicle missing here, namely the C7 right pedicle (**a, b**). The neighbouring bone is normal. The three-dimensional CT scan (**c**) confirms the absence of the pedicle which is an anatomical variant with no pathological significance. In this case, pedicular agenesis is associated with hypoplasia of the posterior tubercle of the transverse process. This is frequently associated with spina bifida. Pedicular agenesis is mostly encountered at C5 or C6.

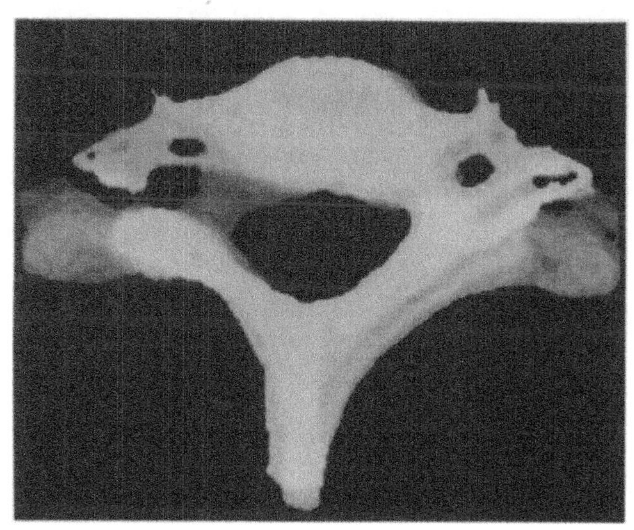

c

17

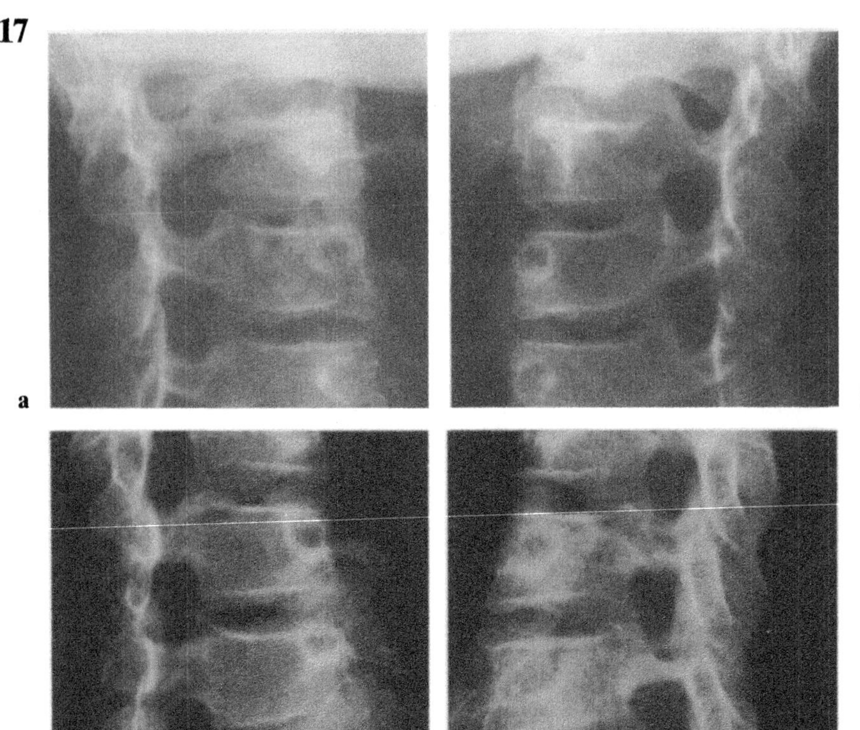

As you know the pedicles well by now, please suggest the diagnosis in these two patients. To assist you, we have localized the areas of interest.

---

b You will have certainly realised that the right C4 pedicle is in the shape of a half-moon or a crescent (**e**). This should have immediately brought to mind the possibility of a dolichovertebral artery. This is confirmed in **a**, where you should have noted an enlargement of the superior part of C3–C4 foramen, but sparing the uncinate processes.

d Part of the cortex of the right C6 pedicle is outlined by a radiolucent line corresponding to a fracture (**f**) which isonly faintly visible in **c**.

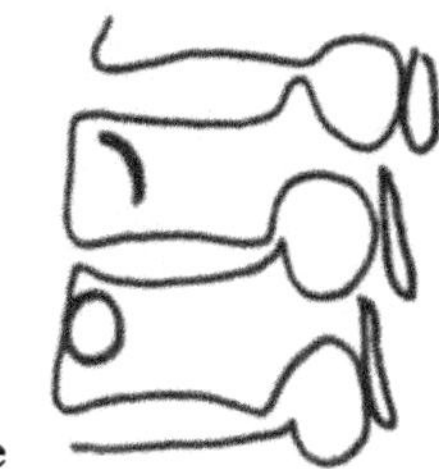

e

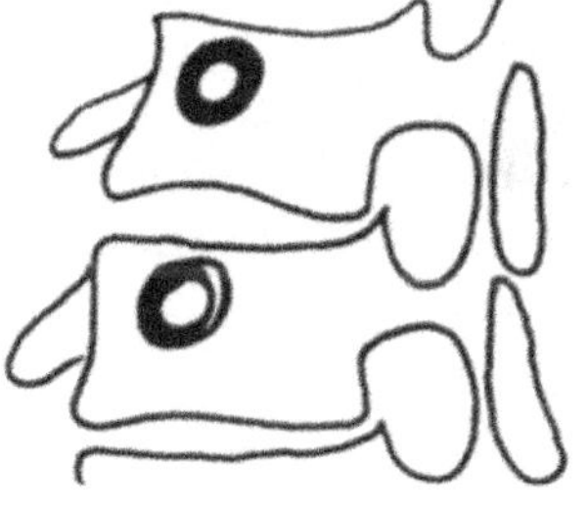

f

18

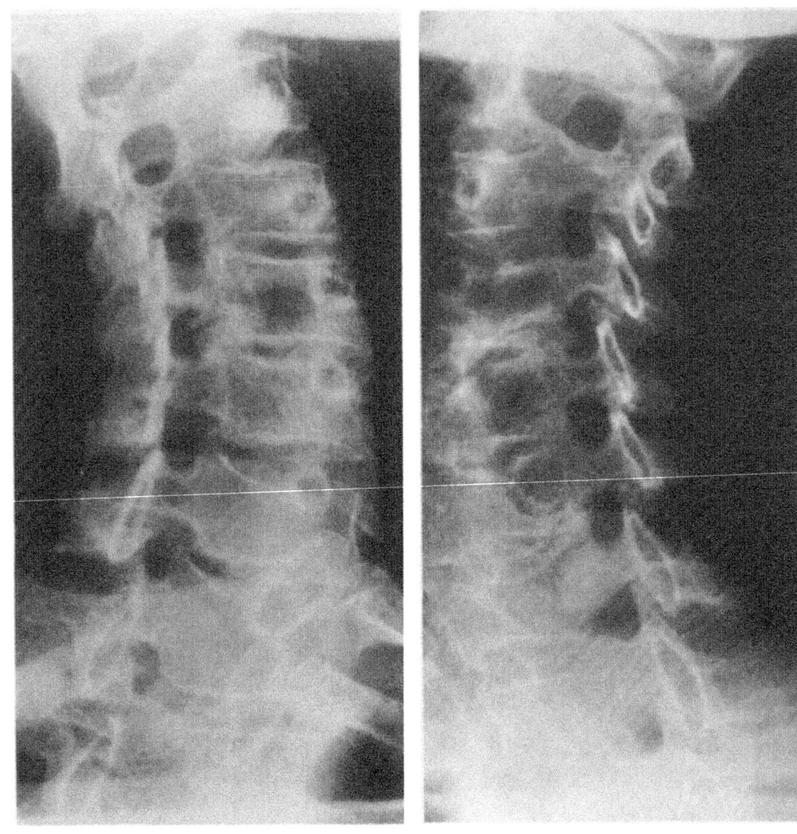

a

Now that the cervical pedicles hold no more secrets for you, what do you think of these radiographs?

There are degenerative changes in the uncinate processes causing a clear narrowing of several intervertebral foramina. Do not spend too much time on these as these observations are often not clinically significant. If you examined the pedicles carefully before looking at the intervertebral foramina, you will have immediately realised that these two radiographs are not of the same patient!

a The left C3 pedicle is condensed (**c**); however, it is normal in **b**.

b The left C7 pedicle is condensed (**d**); however, it is normal in **a** (if the right C5, C6 and C7 pedicles cannot be seen very well in **b**, it is, as is sometimes possible, because they are hidden by the projection of voluminous osteophytes on the vertebral bodies).

In both cases, the diagnosis is, of course, osteoblastic metastasis.

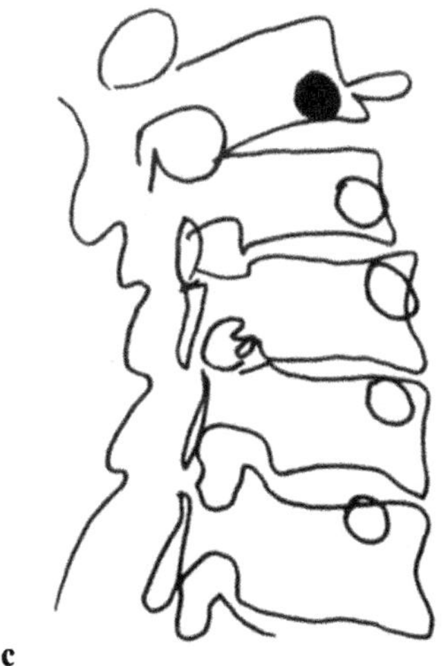

c

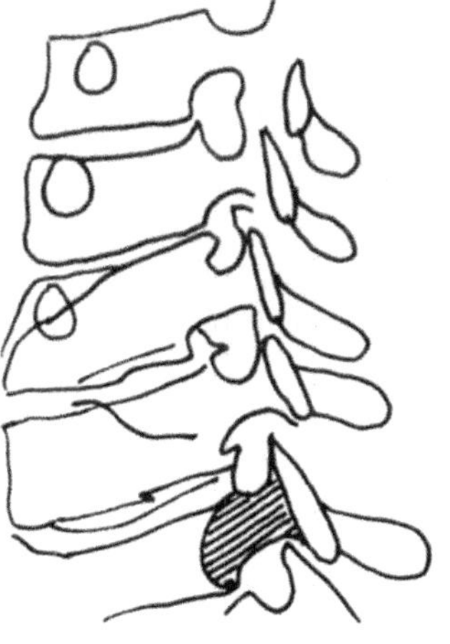

d

19

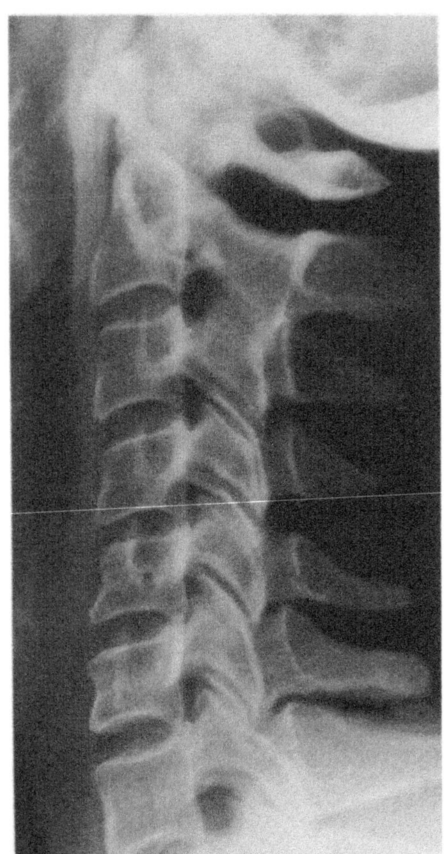

a

Case 19

What do you notice in this lateral radiograph of the cervical spine?

With a few seconds, you should have scanned the prevertebral soft tissues, the alignment of the anterior and posterior margins of the vertebral bodies, the safety space which is clearly visible between the posterior aspect of the articular processes and the spinolaminar line: these are all normal and the visualisation of the intervertebral foramina of C2–C3 and C7–T1 is reassuring (**a**).

However two features have probably struck you: there is an osseous bridge, carrying the vertebral artery, above the posterior arch of C1. This is a common anatomical variant. There is also a small hole projected onto the centre of the body of C5. As shown in the CT scan (**b**), it is a case of an unusually large vascular channel, orientated in the coronal plane, which drains posteriorly through the basivertebral veins into the epidural veins at the posterior margin of the vertebral body. This vascular channel, which is seen more frequently in the lumbar region, is not pathological.

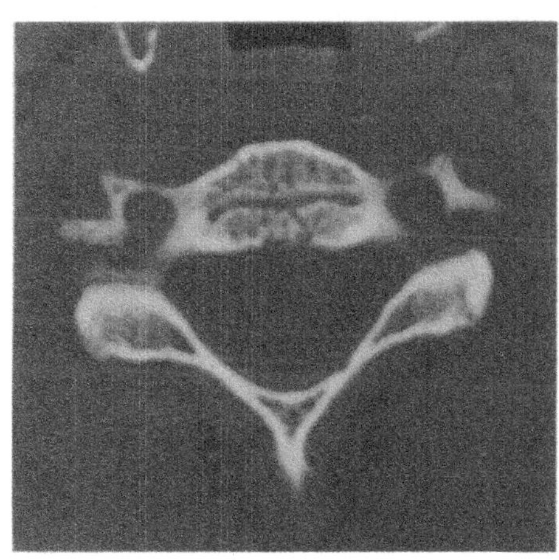

b

20

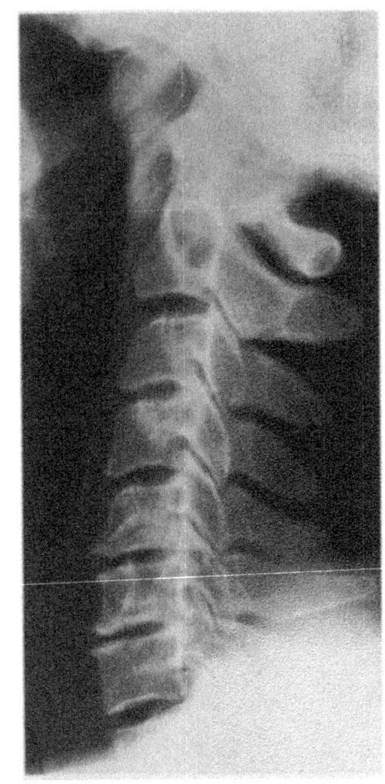

a

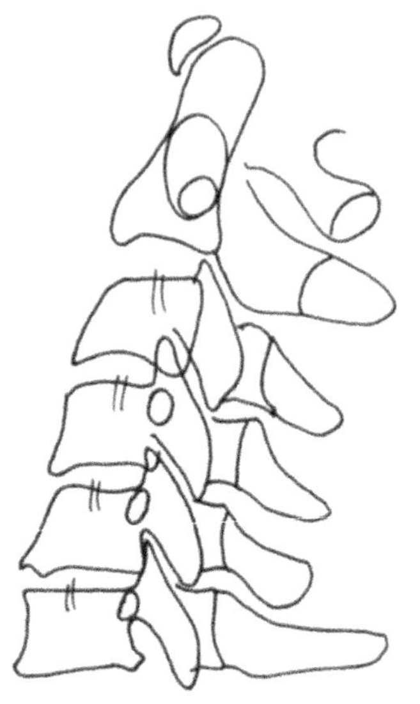

c

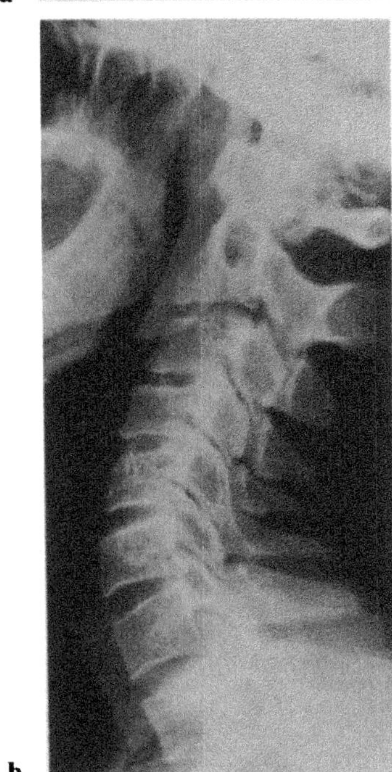

b

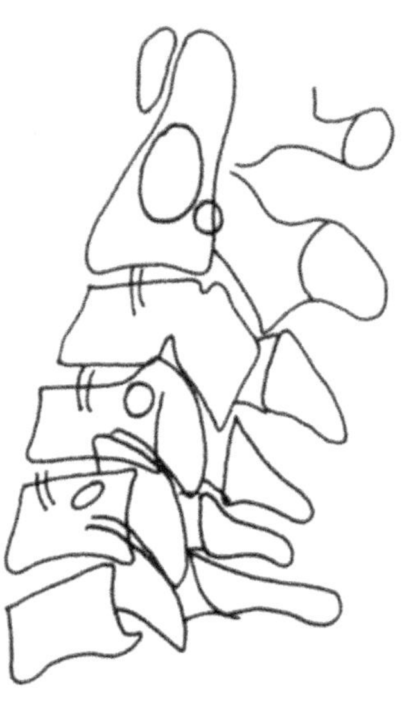

d

There is an eye-like image which catches your attention in each of these lateral radiographs: if you have assimilated all the preceding information, you will easily be able to find the whys and wherefores.

In a systematic analysis of these two radiographs, you will have noted that the articular processes are located more anteriorly than usual: they project onto the posterior part of the vertebral body; for example, look at the superior articular processes of C5 in **b**. This anterior location of the articular processes is responsible for the nonvisualisation of the foramina C2–C3 and C7–T1, which you will have already noted. You will have remembered that this positioning of the articular processes is most often characterised by a reduction in size and particularly a frontalisation of the pedicles, which are then visible "de face" in the lateral view. The pedicles are better visualised when the articular processes are located very anteriorly, for example, the pedicles of C5 in **a** and **b**.

Your attention was called on the other hand by other eye-like images projected this time on C2.

The canal of the vertebral artery, has a horizontal course for a short distance. This canal is perfectly visible in **a** (**c**) and less clearly is **b** (**d**). In addition, we can see a clear, oval and well-defined radiolucent area with a dense margin, known as Harris's ring; it is better visualised in **b** (**d**) than in **a** (**c**). Harris's ring is not a true ring but only an image corresponding to the projection of the insertion of the C2 articular processes in the lateral view. The superior pole of Harris's ring corresponds to the base of the odontoid process. Harris's ring is destroyed in C2 fractures extending below the base of the odontoid process. The visualisation of Harris's ring is not at all uniform; it depends on the form of the C2 articular processes and on the orientation of the X-ray beam.

21

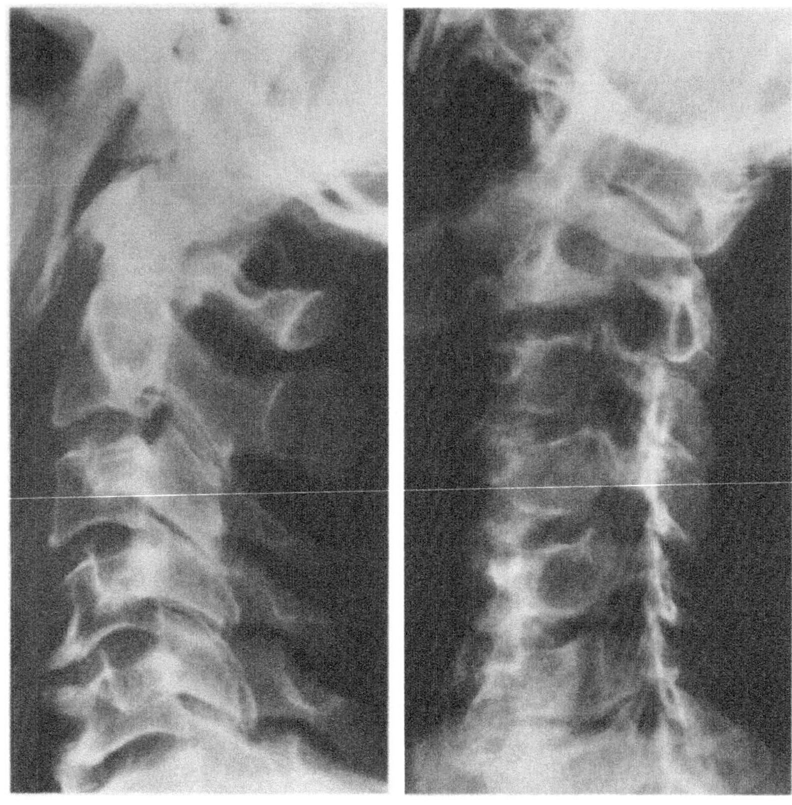

a

Posterior interapophyseal degenerative changes, degenerative changes of the uncinate process with narrowing of the left C6–C7 intervertebral foramen, huge anterior osteophytes (**a**) ..., but what is really a cause for concern is a large lacuna at C5: what is your diagnosis?

It must be noted that this lacuna at C5 is only visualised in one of the two images. It is an artifact caused by the very large osteophytes of the vertebral bodies, anteriorly and laterally, superiorly and inferiorly, defining between them a roughly rounded area (**c**). Note that, in the oblique view (**b**), the density of this pseudolacuna is quite the same as that of the normal bone of the bodies of C3 and C4. On the other hand, the image of the osseous structure marking the margins of the lacuna, especially at the front, is dense owing to the superposition of large osteophytes.

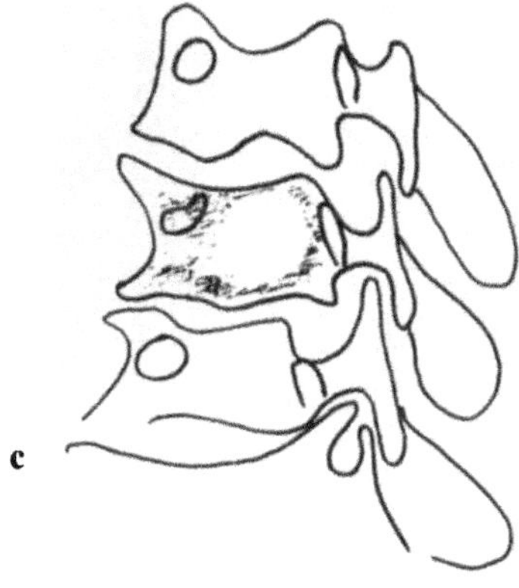
c

22

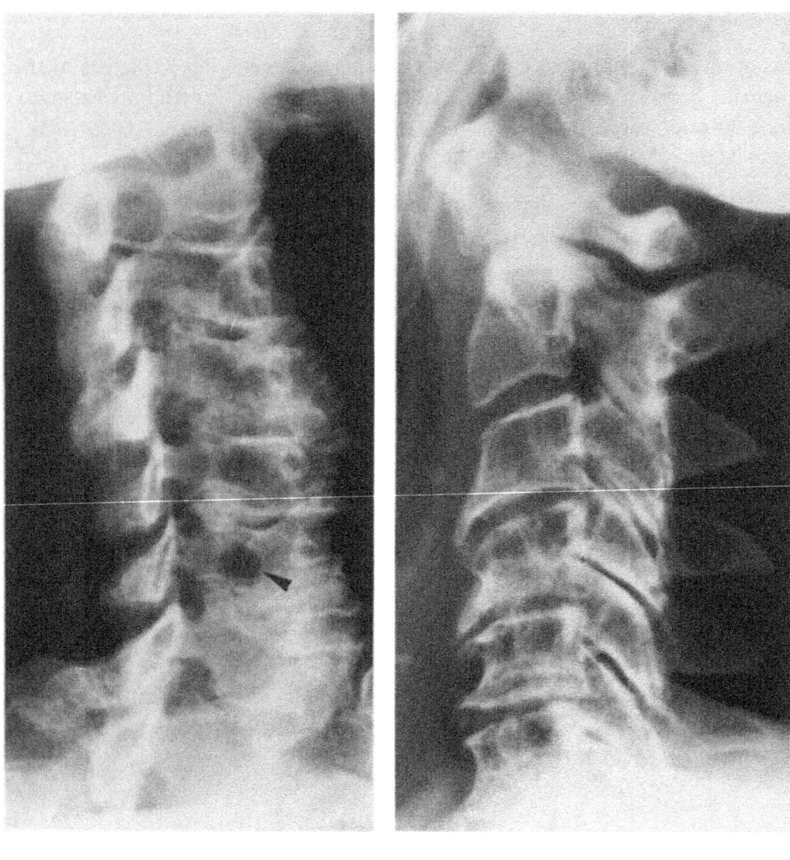

a

In the oblique view, you can see a lacuna-like image on the posterior part of the body of C6 *(arrow)*. Is it a true or a false lacuna?

As shown in **c** and **d**, the lacuna-like image is visualised in both projections: there is therefore little chance of this being an artifact. Moreover, as can be seen in the oblique view (**a**), the bone around the defect is not sclerosed. It is therefore a true osseous lacuna (metastasis?).

If you have made only this one diagnosis, do not rejoice too quickly, because you may have overlooked two other diagnoses which could be of clinical importance. There is an atlanto-odontoid dislocation (**b**) which is narrowing the spinal canal at C1: in this case it is imperative to obtain radiographs during careful flexion of the head to see if the dislocation increases with flexion, as is frequently the case with rheumatoid polyarthritis. In this cases there is a possibility of spinal cord compression.

Moreover, there is a global stenosis of the cervical canal, because the safety space is missing all along the cervical column. This could therefore represent another possible cause of spinal cord compression.

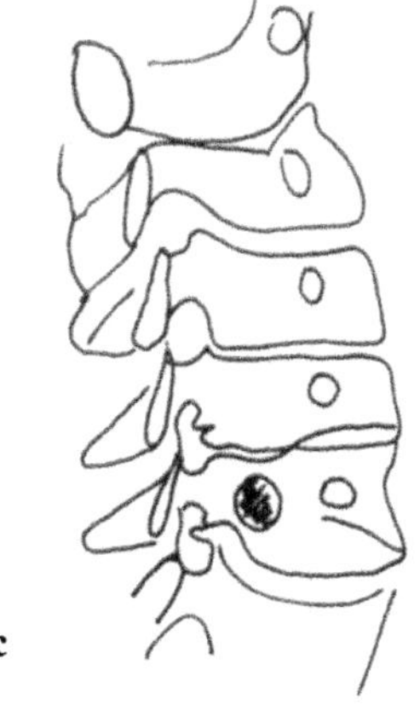
c

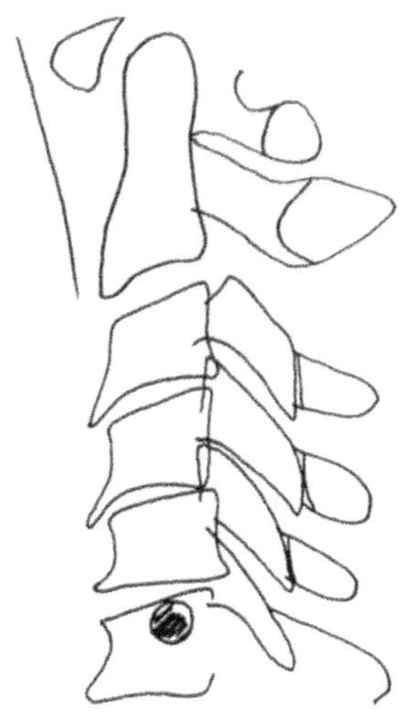
d

23

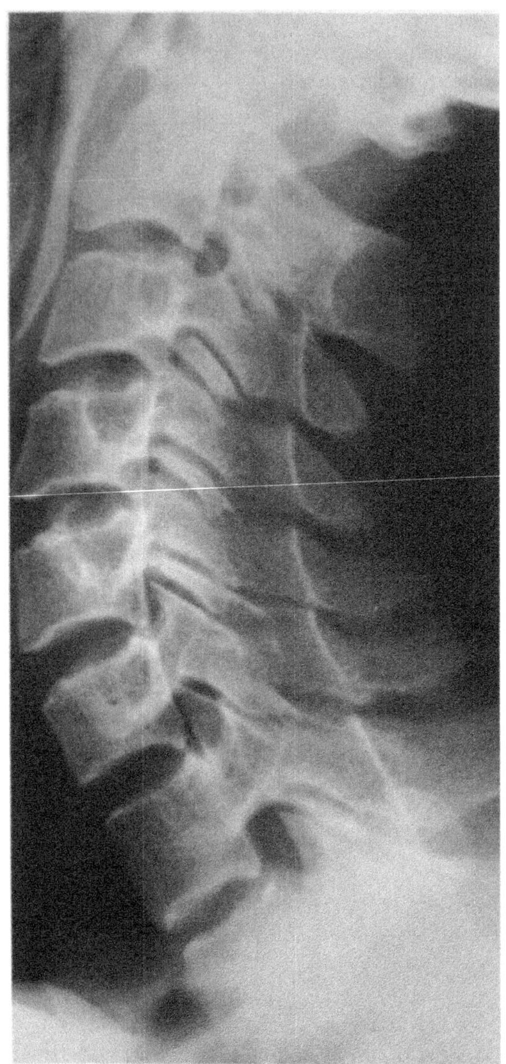

As the previous exercise was a little difficult, I am going to allow you to relax a bit here and even give you the diagnosis: a slowly growing cervical intramedullary tumor. The principal radiological signs are: (a) the anteroposterior diameter of the cervical canal is increased: at more than 20 mm it is greater than the anteroposterior diameter of the vertebral bodies; (b) the safety space is clearly enlarged. (c) The posterior surfaces of the C4 and C5 bodies are concave posteriorly following the general widening of the cervical canal. (d) The spinolaminar line has lost its normal anterior convexity and is straight. But do not go on to the next exercise without answering the following question: what has happened to the posterior surfaces of the articular processes of C3, C4 and C5?

Look back at any figure of a cervical vertebra, for example the figure shown on page 1. Normally, in the lateral view, the posterior surfaces of the articular processes are exactly tangential to the X-ray beam. Therefore, radiologically, they almost always appear to have a dense margin. If the spinal canal is much enlarged and rounded, the orientation of the articular processes may be modified: in the lateral view, the posterior surfaces of the articular processes are therefore oblique in relation to the X-ray beam and are thus not clearly defined.

24

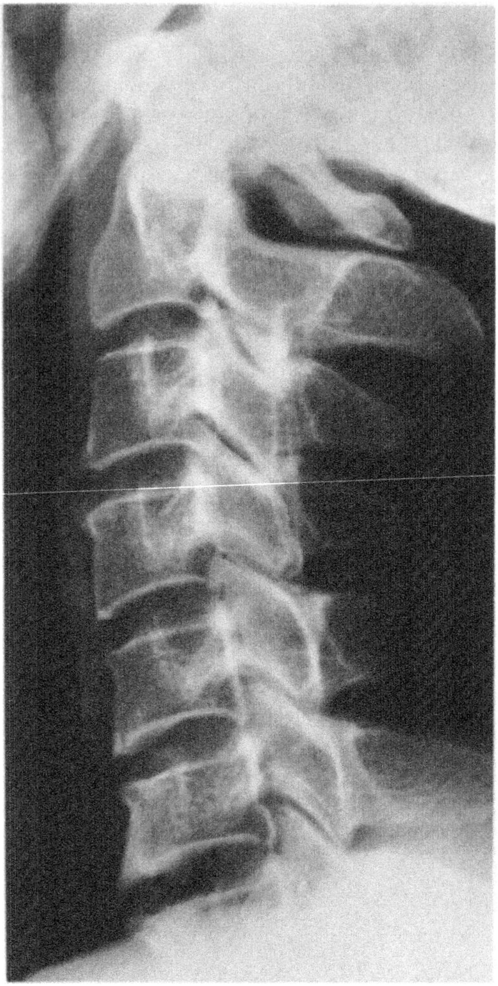

a

In this case, what do you think of the cervico-occipital junction?

Whatever the question is, your analysis should be systematic. Therefore you will have not missed noticing stenosis of the canal as the safety space is practically nonexistant below C3 (**a, b**). If there is spinal stenosis, the subarachnoid spaces are narrow, and the spinal cord is not well protected in case of compression due to traumatism or posterior osteophytosis of the vertebral bodies.

In fact, the answer to the question should have been that there is a congenital anomaly of the posterior arch of atlas. One half of the posterior arch of the atlas appears to be free and is not fused with its counterpart. This is a minor anatomical variant.

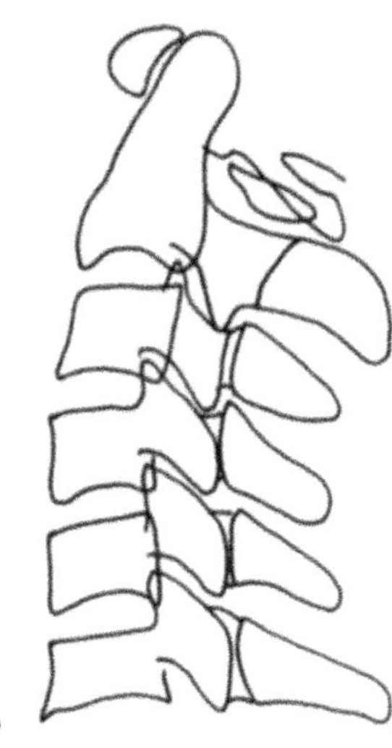

b

25

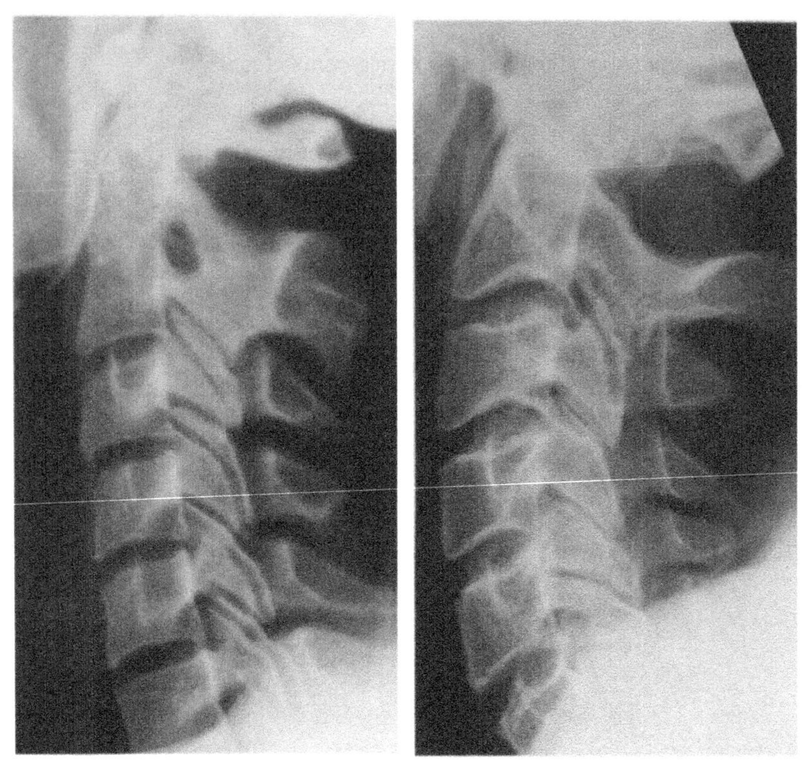

a

What makes these two lateral radiographs similar?

Many things!

a You will have noted a congenital fusion of C2 and C3. The spinolaminar line from C2 to C6 is straight, indicating local compression. However, the spinal canal is not really enlarged; but the safety space, which is also not enlarged, presents an abnormal radiolucency, particularly at C3–C5: this abnormal radiolucency of the laminae, together with the straightened spinolaminar line indicates long-standing increased intraspinal pressure, which, in this case, was due to a spinal cord astrocytoma. Fusion of C2 and C3 is a minor independent malformation.

b In this case also, there is an osseous abnormality: partial occipitalisation of the atlas. In other respects, the cervical canal is enlarged as indicated by the increased anteroposterior size of the safety space. Here, too, the laminae are very radiolucent because they are so thin, which can be seen very well in the CT scan (**c**). Again, note the absence of the normal convexity of the spinolaminar line. This is a case of syringomyelia associated with a Chiari malformation and occipitalisation of the atlas. Note that importance cannot be attached to the thickness of the soft tissues in front of C2 in cases of occipitalisation of the atlas or basilar impression.

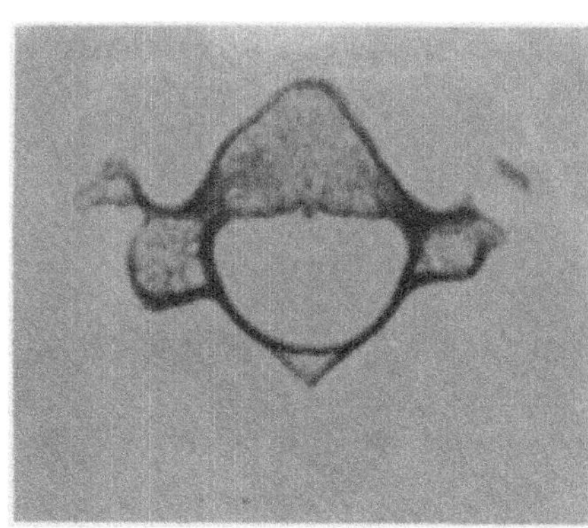

c

26

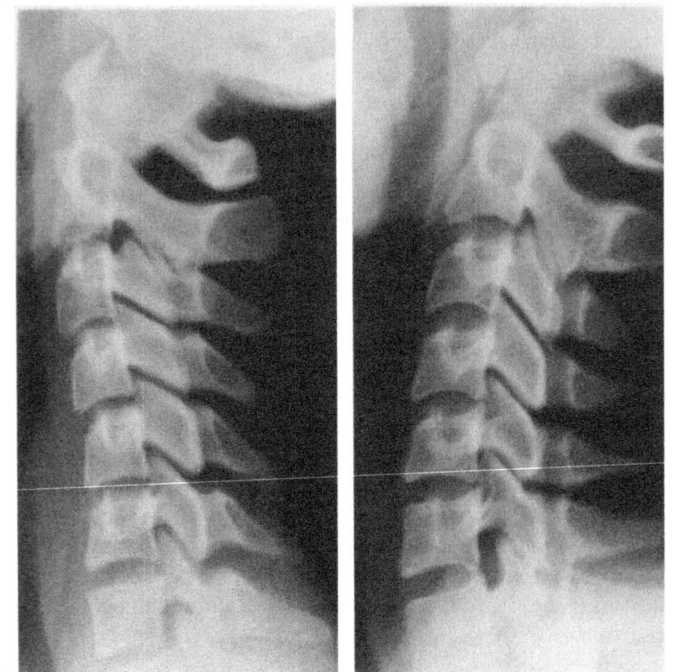

a b

a This patient is a 14-year-old girl in whom the vertebral ring apophyses have begun to fuse with the bodies.

b In this 17-year-old girl, the ring apophyses have fused with the vertebral bodies.

The two girls have something in common, but are different in other respects. What do you think?

---

a The posterior surface of the articular process of C6 has a horn-shaped tubercle directed posterosuperiorly and projected onto the safety space. This osseous beak is an anatomical variant which is sometimes present at C6, most often unilaterally, and is the result of hypertrophy of the insertion tubercle of the semispinalis capitis. It can be seen very well in the three-dimensional CT scan (**c**).

This osseous spine may be present at two levels, at C5 and at C6 as in **b**, but the osseous horns in these cases are less prominent.

These anatomical variants should have drawn your attention as they project onto the safety space, the study of which should form part of a systematic analysis of the cervical spine.

Finally, have you noted unusual visualisation of the C6–C7 foramen in **b**? C7 presents all the signs of thoracisation, including a cervical rib.

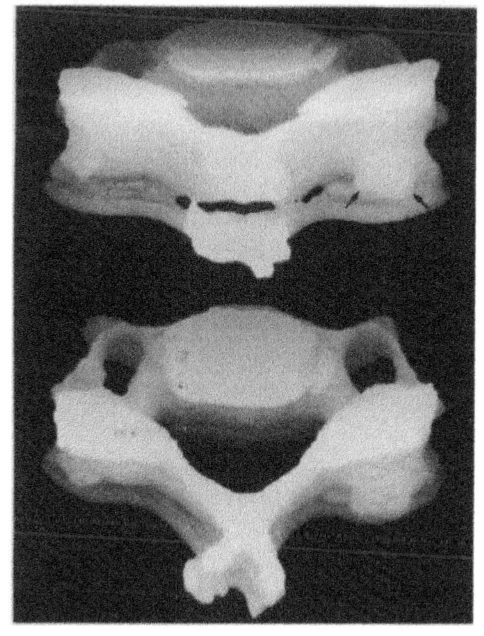

27

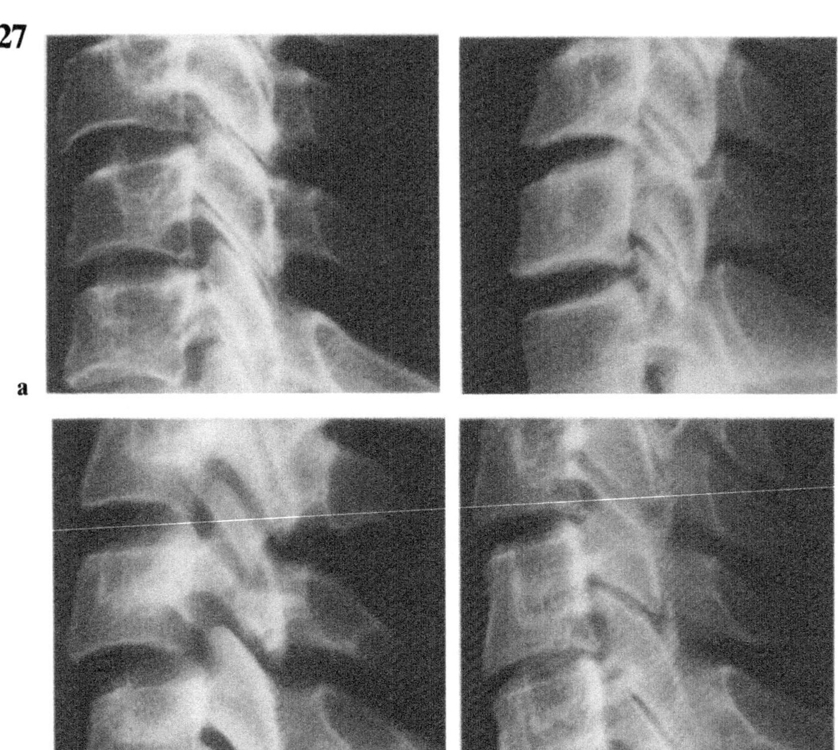

a

c

In **a–d** there are four osseous “beaks” projecting from the posterior aspect of the articular processes onto the safety space. Only one of these represents a hypertrophy of the insertion tubercle of the semispinalis capitis. Which one?

The correct response is **b**: this image is typical of the insertion tubercle of the semispinalis capitis: this extensor muscle of the head maintains the equilibrium of the head and also plays a role in the rotation of the head. This anatomical variant has to be distinguished from an osseous spur which is often present in cases of posterior interapophyseal degenerative changes (**a** and **e**).

c There is a fracture of the articular mass with displacement of the inferior articular process which is projected onto the safety space.

Finally, in **d**, the beak-like image is an artifact: the posterior surfaces of the right and left C6 articular processes are not superimposed and even appear separated as a result of the angle of the X-ray beam.

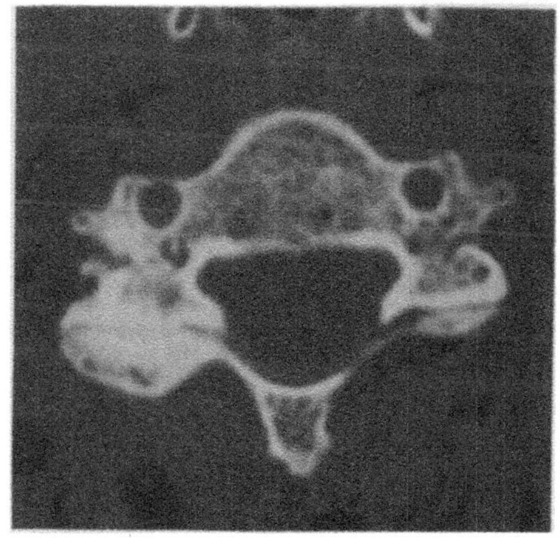

e

28

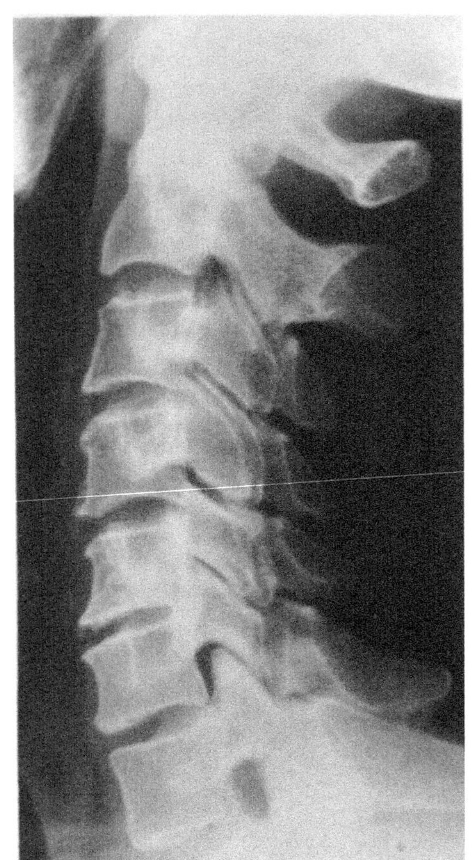

a

This radiograph (**a**) was taken following an injury. What is your diagnosis?

Above C5 there is a slight rotation of the vertebral bodies as shown by the doubled lines of the posterior surfaces of the vertebral bodies and the articular processes.

This rotation of the cervical spine is due to a lesion of the posterior arch of C6: the three-dimensional CT scan (**b**) shows a fracture of the posterior arch at the junction of the lamina and the articular process.

Even small rotation of the vertebral bodies, such as the one here, should make a scrupulous search for a fracture of the posterior arch imperative.

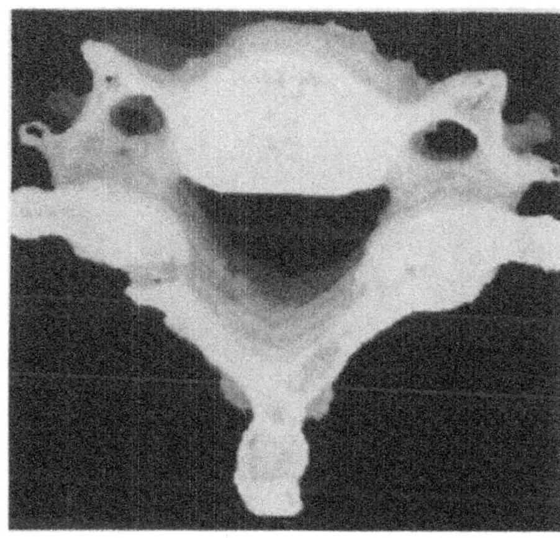

b

29

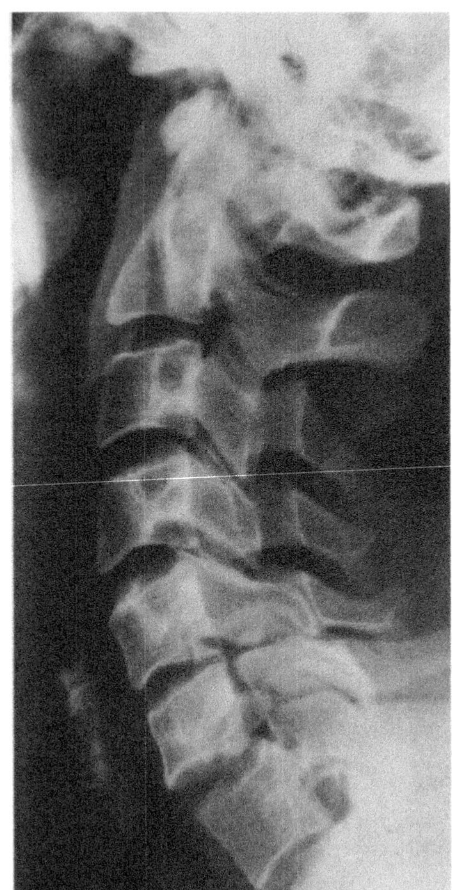

a

This is a case of post-traumatic cervical pain. What do you think?

There is a dysplasia of the C5 and C6 bodies and a congenital anomaly of the posterior arches: your attention will have immediately been drawn by the absence of the safety space at C5 and C6 (**a**). At C5 the articular process is elongated anteroposteriorly; at C6 there is a linear defect posterior to the vertebral body, and the articular process is located more posteriorly than usual. The CT scans (**b** and **c**) confirm the spondylolysis of C6, associated with spina bifida. The diagnosis is therefore a congenital malformation; there is no traumatic lesion.

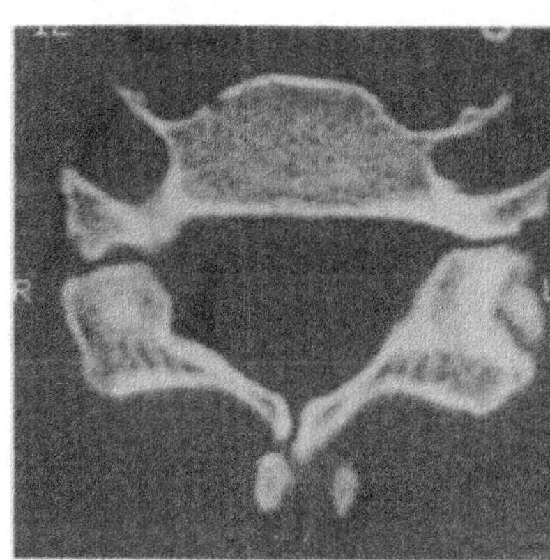

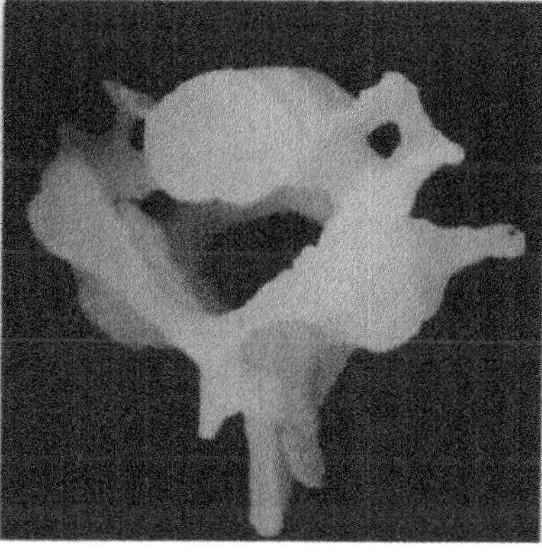

c

30

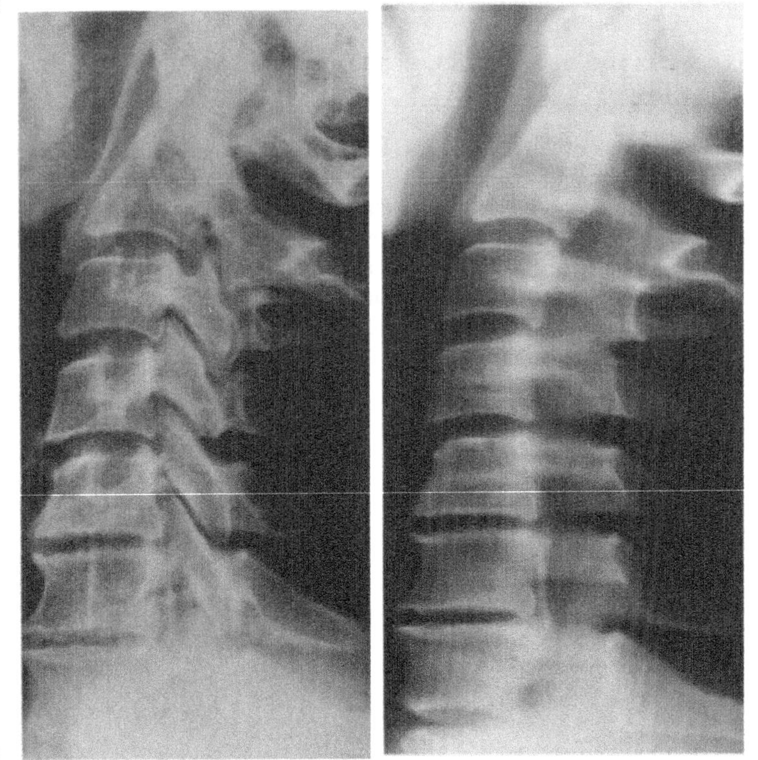

a b

The diagnosis is easy in this case. But can you say what the orientation of the X-ray beam is on the tomogram?

The diagnosis is obviously ossification of the posterior longitudinal ligament. This disease was initially described in the Japanese in whom it is not rare. It is usually located between C3 and C6 (**a–c**). Generally, this dense, calcified band is situated in contact with the posterior surface of the vertebral bodies, but it may be separated from it by a radiolucent space, as is the case here behind C6. Anatomically, these calcifications are situated between the dura mater and the posterior longitudinal ligament. If the ossification is sufficiently thick, it may produce a narrowing of the anteroposterior diameter of the cervical canal causing spinal cord compression.

On the other hand, you will have noticed a well-defined and finely encircled osseous lacuna, in the spinous process of C3, presenting all the characteristics of a benign osseous tumour.

The tomogram was taken perpendicular to the major axis (**b**) of the cervical spine; this point may be important in the tomographic study of the spine which will be discussed later.

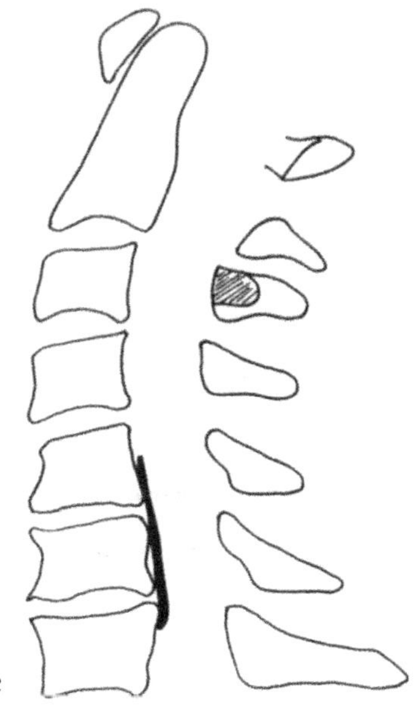

31

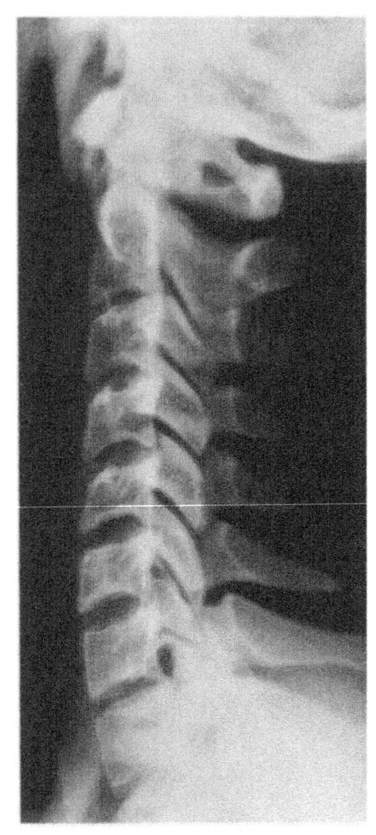

a

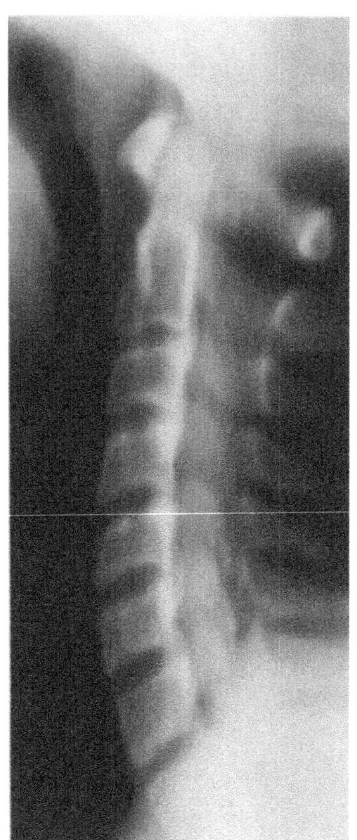

b

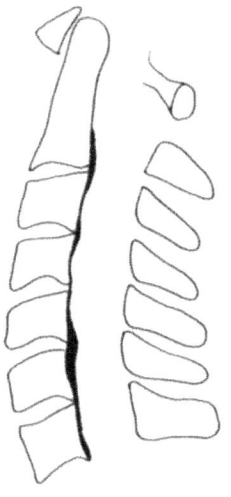

Is this ossification of the posterior longitudinal ligament (**a, b**)?

No. You will have noted that the tomogram was obtained with a beam parallel to the axis of the spine. This has accentuated the projection of the vertebral unci which are particularly prominent here and directed partly cephalad and partly posteriorly, as can be seen in the CT scan (**c**).

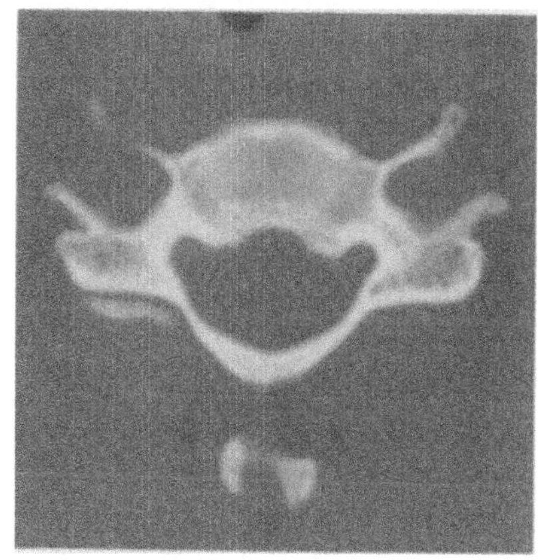

c

32

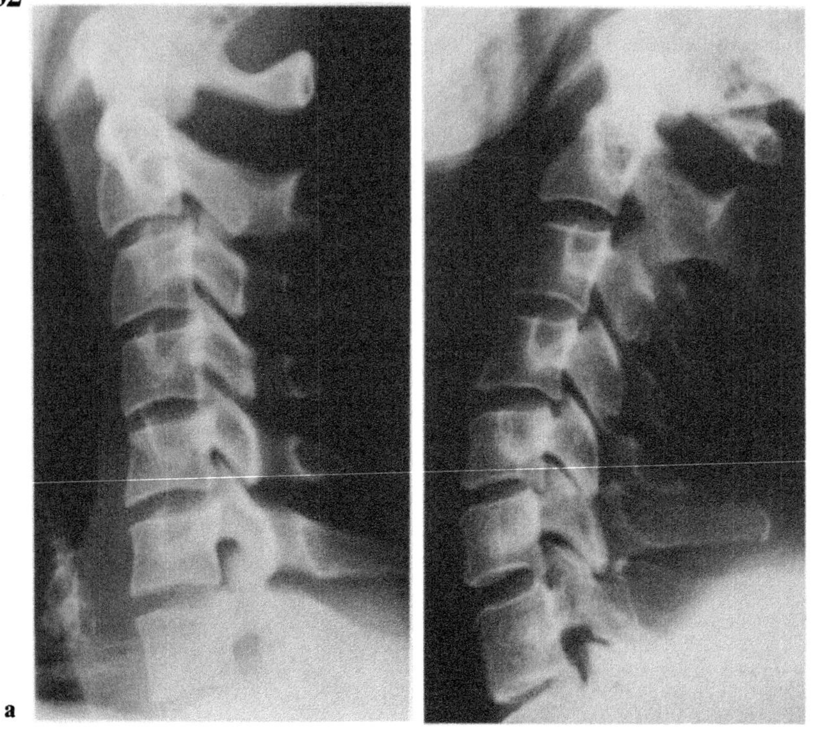

By now you are used to observe carefully a number of features on lateral radiographs of the cervical spine: the prevertebral soft tissues, the safety space and the spinolaminar line. Do not forget them, we shall soon need them again. Now consider another essential feature: the posterior surfaces of the vertebral bodies. What do you think of the two radiographs shown here?

---

a You will have already recognised hypertrophy of the uncus, particularly at C5. There is no vertebral misalignment here: the posterior spinolaminar line is perfectly aligned.

b There is retrolisthesis of C5 which is admittedly less than 2 mm, but it is still very important to recognise it. The posterior displacement of the spinolaminar line at C5 in relation to C6 would confirm vertebral displacement if necessary. On closer inspection, you will find, at the superior part of the C5–C6 intervertebral disc space, a small gasseous radiolucency indicating a discal lesion (**c**). These extremely subtle radiological signs may, however, signify major lesions in the discs or ligaments, as demonstrated in the diagram (**d**) of a radiograph taken in flexion (not shown). Here one can see: an angulation at C5–C6 with spondylolisthesis of C5, indicating a lesion of the disc and the anterior longitudinal ligament; a dislocation of the articular processes of C5–C6 indicating a tear of the articular capsule; and an abnormal space between the laminae and the spinous processes of C5 and C6 indicating a tear of the ligamenta flava and the interspinous ligaments. This is a severe cervical strain, necessitating surgical management. All cases of vertebral misalignment, even minimal ones, should be examined carefully and the possibility of a discoligamentous lesion should be considered.

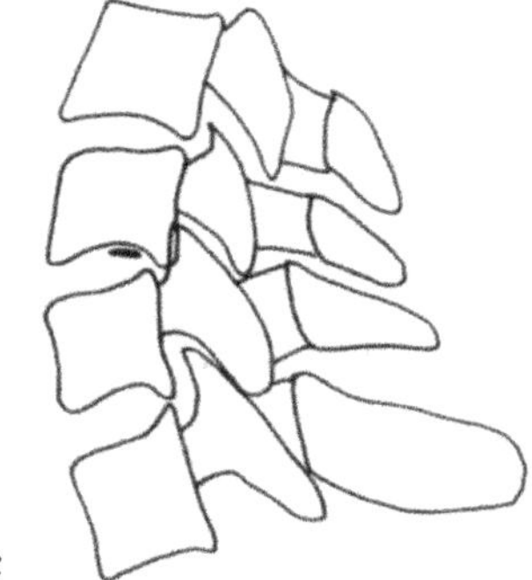

c

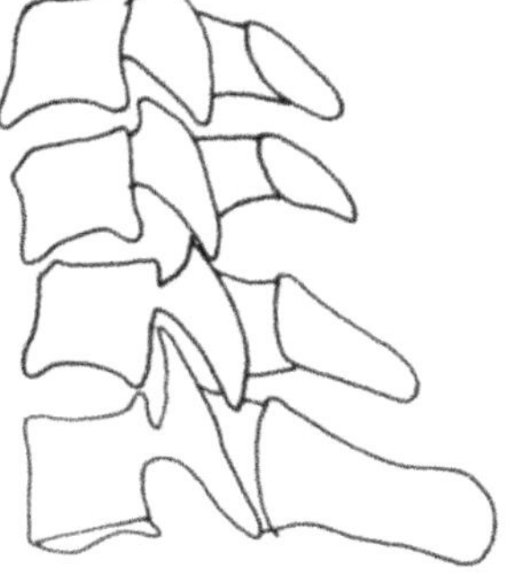

d

33

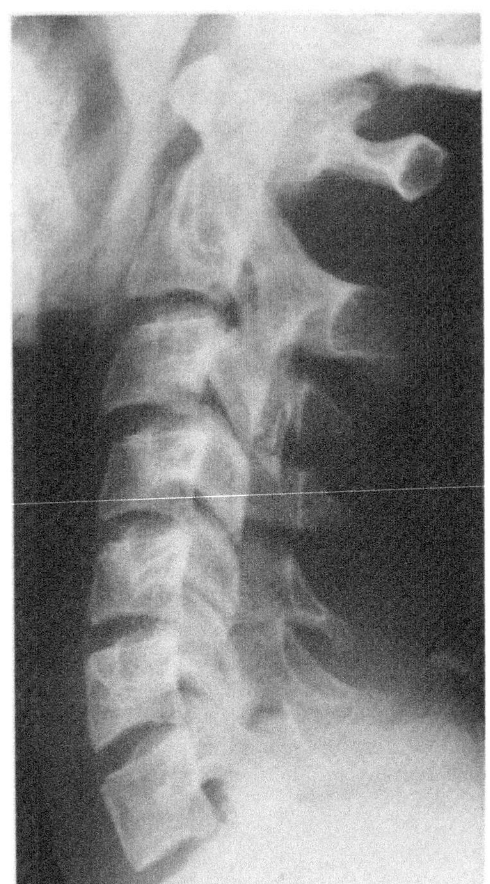

a

Is this hypertrophy of the C4 uncus? Or a true vertebral slippage? Or a C1–C2 dislocation?

The existence of a small V-shaped space between the anterior surface of the odontoid process and the anterior arch of atlas constitutes an anatomical variant which is frequently seen, particularly in young patients and with flexion of the head (**b**). On the other hand, a space between C1 and C2, even if it is narrow, should always be regarded with suspicion if it has parallel sides.

There is spondylolisthesis of C3: the body of C3 has slipped forward in relation to C4 (**a**), as indicated by the anterior displacement of the spinolaminar line of C3. Above all, there is a fracture of the C3 articular process, which has slipped posteriorly, projecting onto the safety space (**c**). There is slight physiological hypertrophy of the C4 uncus.

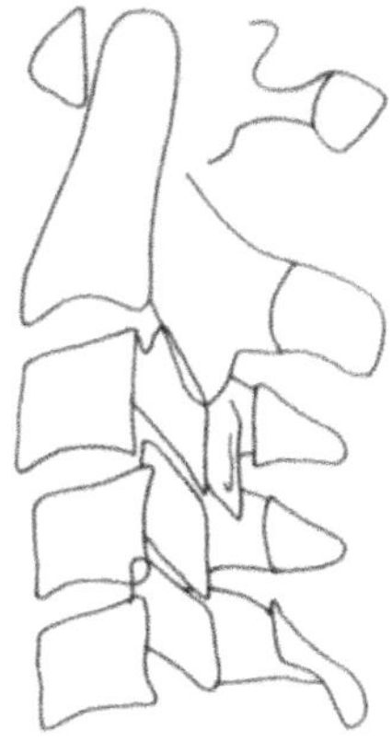

b

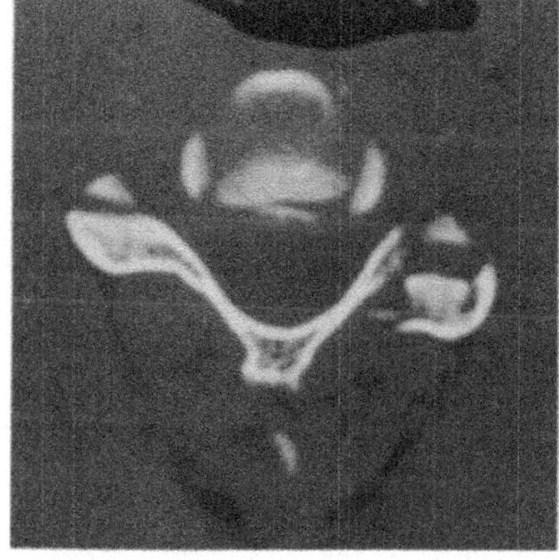

c

34

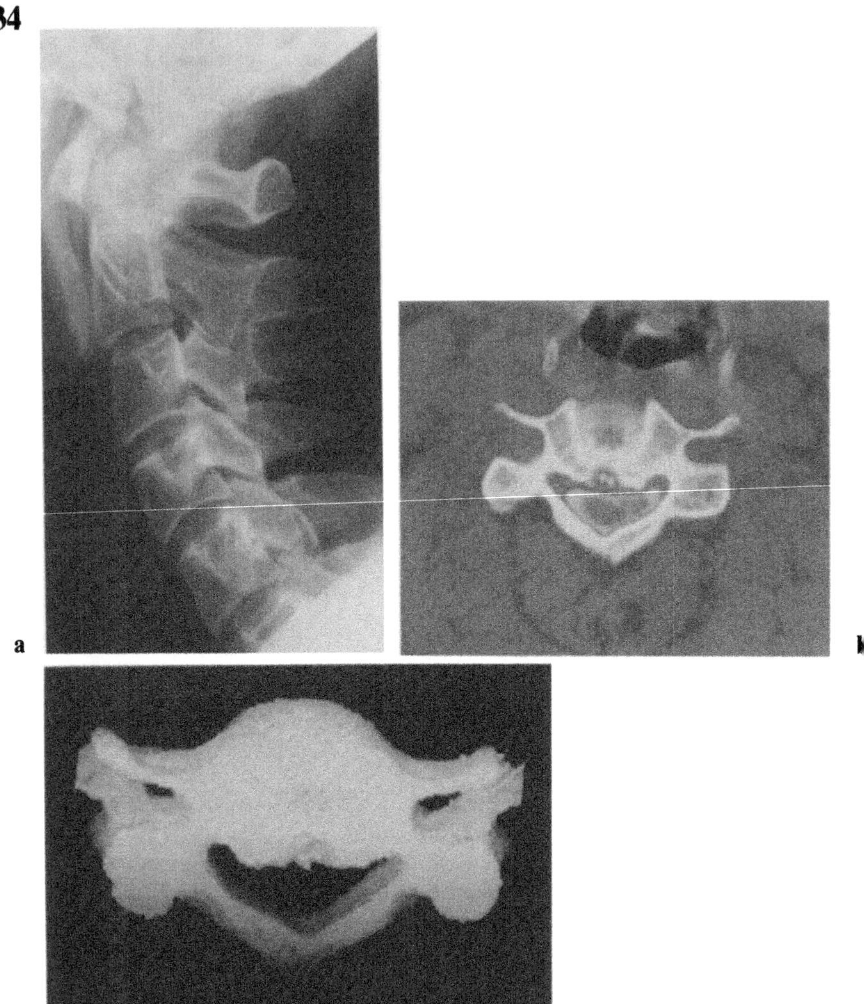

These radiographs are from a patient suspected of having spinal cord compression. What do you think?

If you have examined the posterior surfaces of the vertebral bodies, you will have noticed an abnormal bulge on the posterior surface of C4, resulting in a local narrowing of the spinal canal (**a, d**).

The axial CT scan, performed after subarachanoid contrast injection (**b**), and the three-dimensional CT scan (**c**) confirm that the body of C4 is asymmetric and is bulging posteriorly, giving rise to unilateral narrowing of the canal with ipsilateral spinal cord compression. This is not a case of degenerative spinal stenosis, but a congenital anomaly of the C4 vertebral body.

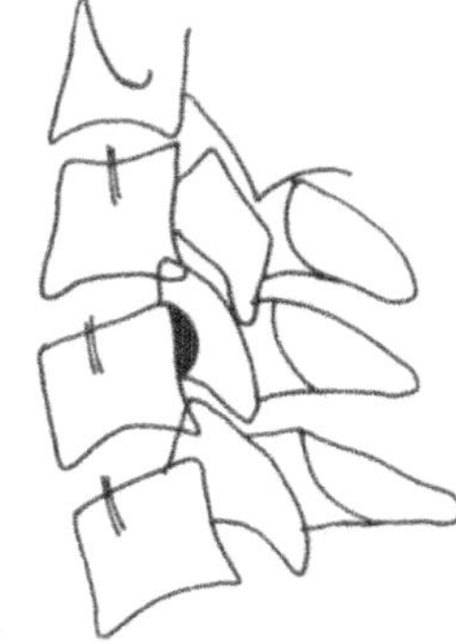

d

35

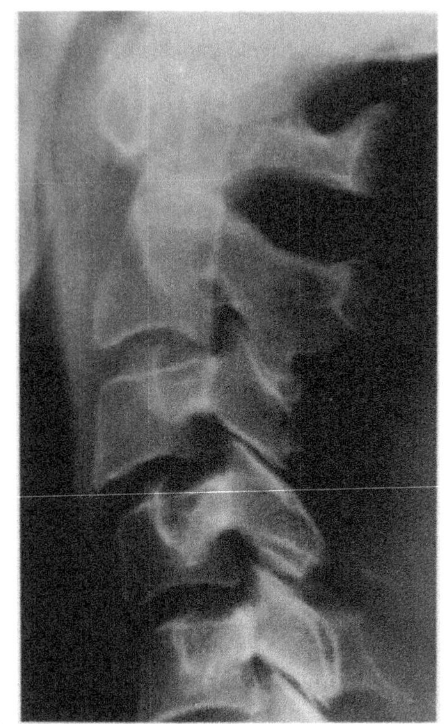

a

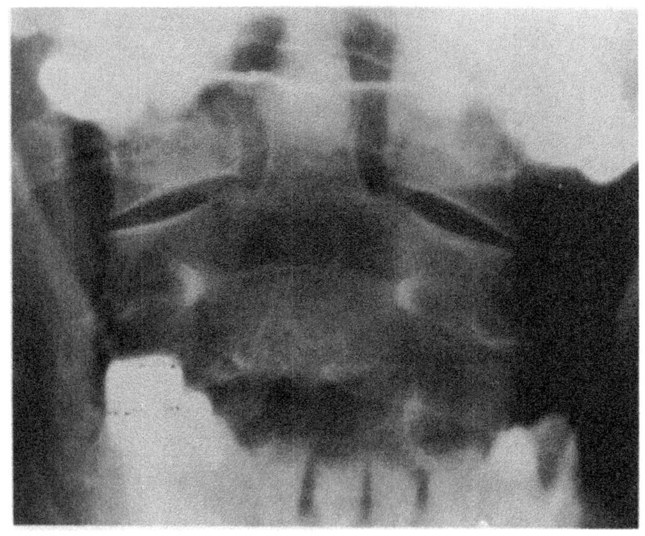

b

Case 35 **35**

This patient had post-traumatic cervical pain. What is your diagnosis?

In cases of trauma, the possibility of a fracture of the odontoid process should be constantly kept in mind. This type of fracture is often invisible in the lateral view as well as in the frontal view (**a, b**). It is in these cases that examination of the prevertebral soft tissues is of great value. In this case, the soft tissues in front of C2 are thicker than the anteroposterior diameter of the odontoid process (see case 4, fig. c). The diagram (**c**) is a drawing of a following radiograph obtained some days after the trauma: the diagnosis is easy because the fragments are now displaced.

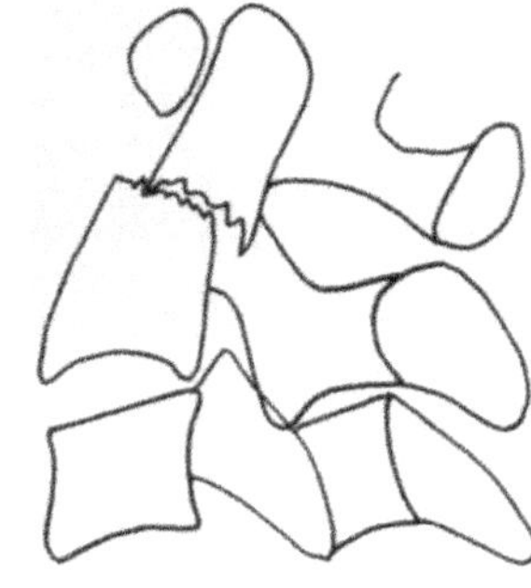

c

36

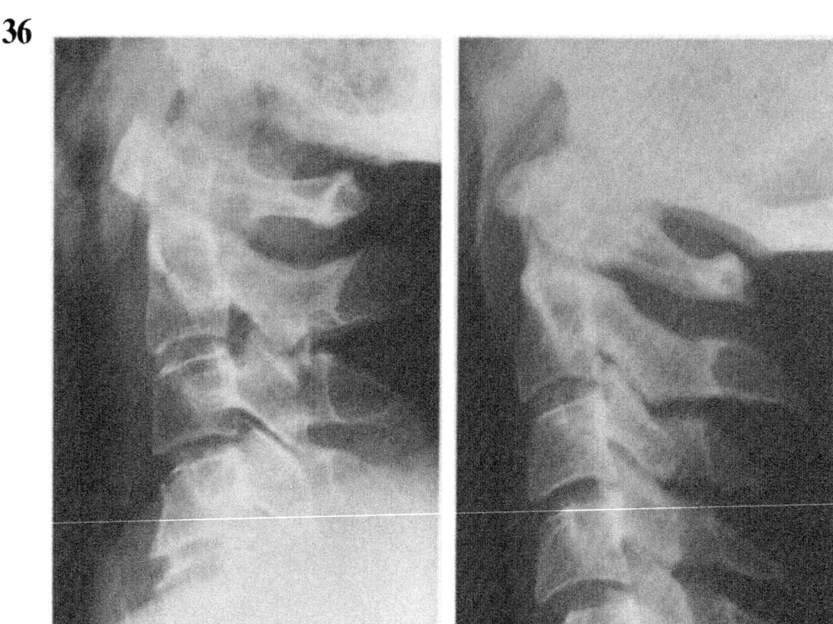

a

Again, there was cervical pain in these two patients following a road traffic accident...

---

a The fracture of C2 is obvious: there is a slight horizontal fracture across the body of C2, extending obliquely superiorly and posteriorly to the pedicle. If you had not seen this fracture, two other signs should have drawn your attention: Harris's ring is broken anteriorly (**c**). Without being really enlarged, the prevertebral soft tissues in front of C2 are convex anteriorly, which is abnormal.

Finally, you may have noted a retrolisthesis of C4: there is in fact minimal malalignment between C4 and C5. At the same level, the height of the intervertebral disc is reduced, and there are osteophytes on the vertebral end-plates. This is a case of degenerative retrolisthesis.

When present, degenerative *retrolisthesis* generally appears *at the same level* as disc degeneration. On the other hand, degenerative *spondylolisthesis,* when present, is generally situated *above* a degenerative disc. These points may be useful in cases of trauma in a degenerative cervical spine. This will be discussed to again later.

b The convexity of the prevertebral soft tissues in front of the base of the odontoid process should make one suspect a fracture of the base of the odontoid process. In this case, the fracture was confirmed by the tomograms.

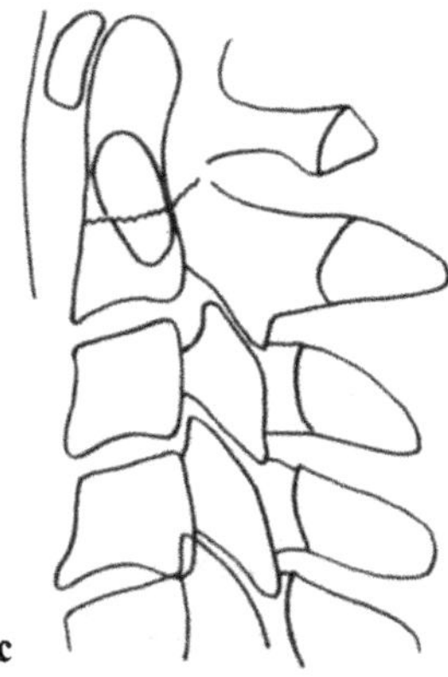

c

37

a

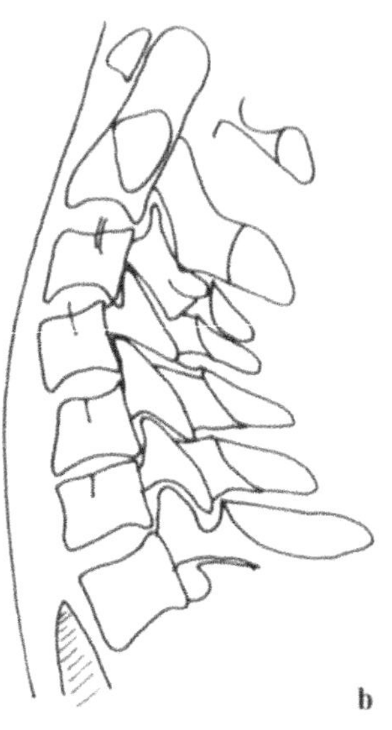

b

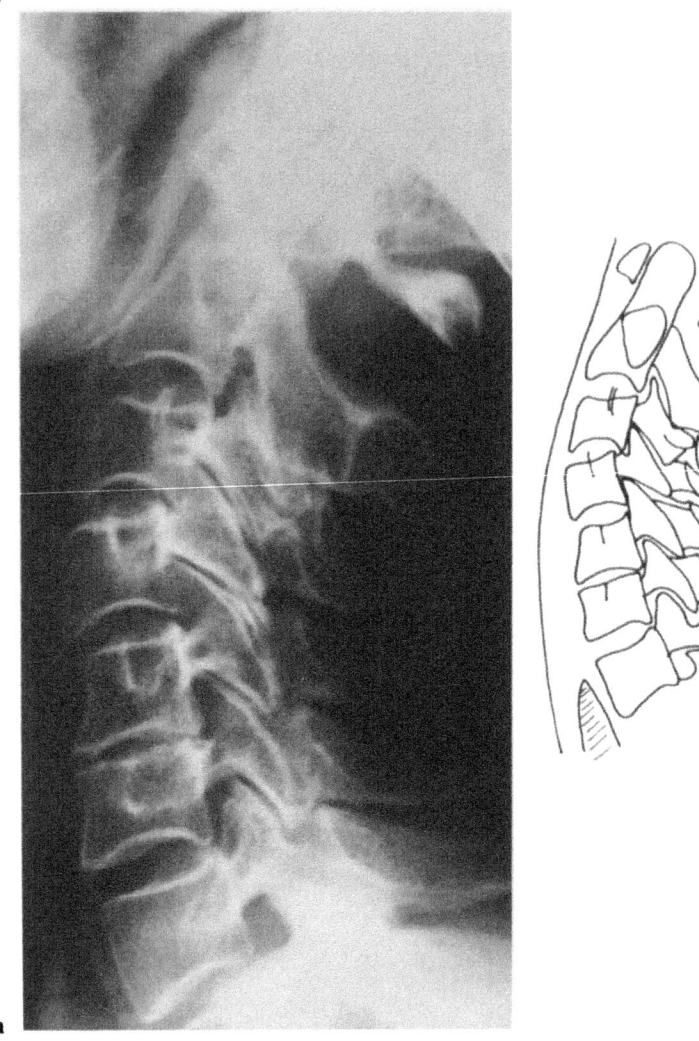

In this case, C3 and C4 are not aligned. Is it spondylolisthesis or retrolisthesis? What is the cause of the malalignment? Have you noticed anything else? What is the significance of the triangular air shadow seen in front of C7?

When two vertebrae are not aligned, the direction of the displacement is given by the direction of the upper one: here, for example, there is malalignment of C3 and C4 (**a, b**). It is a case of retrolisthesis of C3: the posterior aspect of C3 is displaced posteriorly, as is the spinolaminar line, with respect to the corresponding elements of C4. It should also be remembered that retrolisthesis corresponds to the displacement of the vertebra in such a way that the head is drawn backwards, while spondylolisthesis leads to an inverse movement of the head.

In this case, the retrolisthesis is not associated with a discal lesion, but with degenerative changes of the posterior interapophyseal joints. Frequently, this type of posterior interapophyseal degenerative arthritis of the upper cervical spine is secondary to cervical hyperlordosis, which may itself be secondary to dorsal hyperkyphosis.

Incidentally, there are also degenerative changes at C5–C6, with a reduction in height of the intervertebral disc and moderate osteophytes of the vertebral end-plates. You will have also noted a notch on the posterior articular process of C7; this is frequent at this level and indicates, for some, a tendency to C7 thoracisation.

Finally, there is air in the upper part of the oesophagus: in normal subjects, the walls of oesophagus are usually collapsed in the cervical region, but an opening of the lumen of the oesophagus may be observed depending on the respiration time, as is the case here. In other cases, such as in sclerodermia, the anomalies of the oesophageal musculature explain the permanent opening of the oesophagus.

38

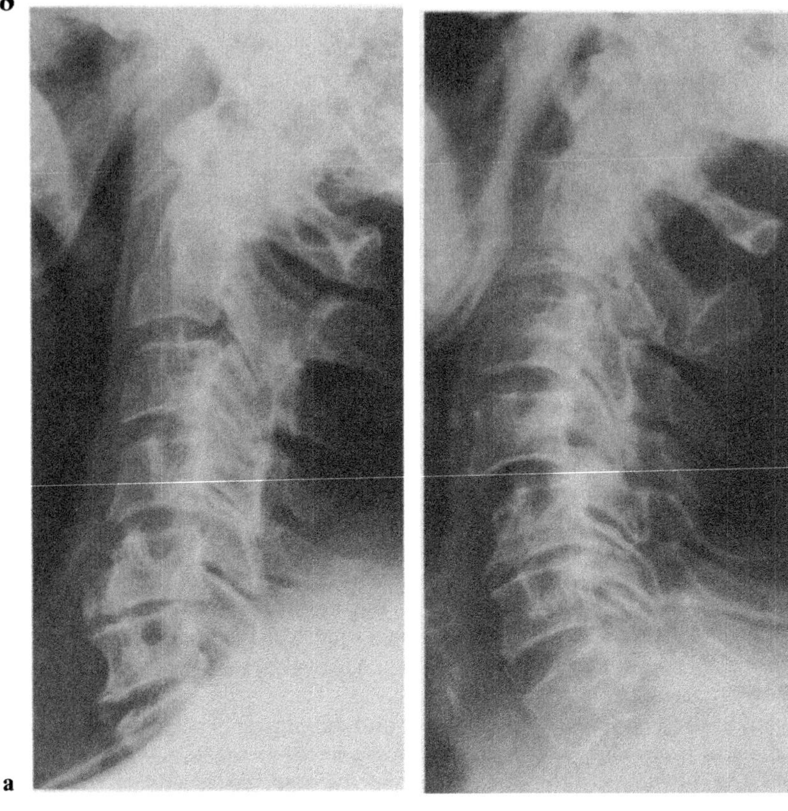

a b

These two radiographs of the cervical spine were obtained after a road traffic accident. There is slippage of some of the vertebral bodies. What do you think?

---

a There is retrolisthesis of C5 above degenerative changes at C5–C6; note the absence of interapophyseal degenerative changes at C5–C6. The prevertebral soft tissues are normal. This C5 retrolisthesis is definitely of a degenerative origin; there is no sign of a traumatic lesion.

b Here, there is also slight retrolisthesis of C5 at the level of the degenerative changes at C5–C6 with no posterior interapophyseal degenerative changes. However, there is also spondylolisthesis of C4 above a disc of normal size: all of these signs are in favour of a degenerative origin of the displacement; the prevertebral soft tissues are also normal.

It must be remembered that retrolisthesis, if it is of a degenerative origin, mostly appears at the same level as the degenerative disc and it is not usually associated with posterior interapophyseal degenerative disease at the level of the displacement; on the other hand, degenerative spondylolisthesis occurs one level above a compressed collapsed degenerative disc and is generally concomitant with interapophyseal degenerative changes at the level of the displacement. The existence of spondylolisthesis or retrolisthesis without these characteristic features should make one immediately suspect a traumatic origin, which will often be confirmed by the presence of a fracture of an articular process and/or by thickening of the prevertebral soft tissues.

39

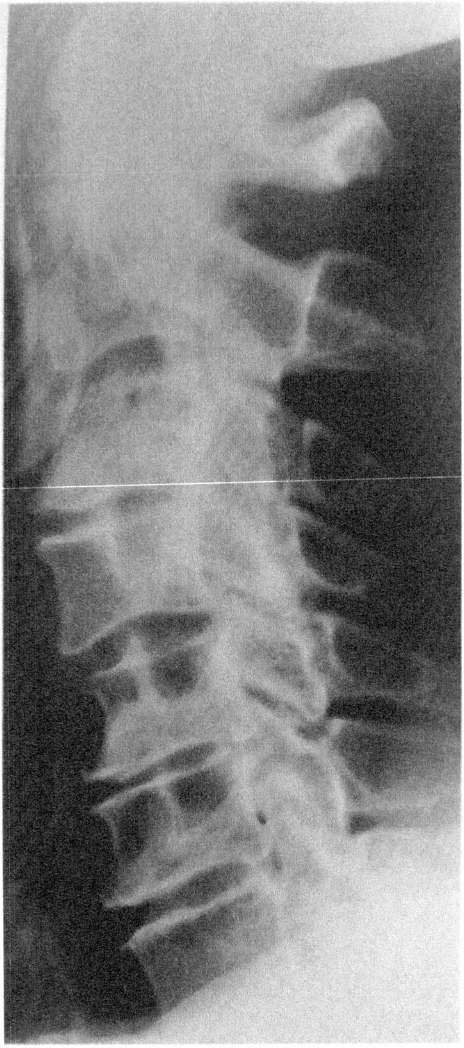

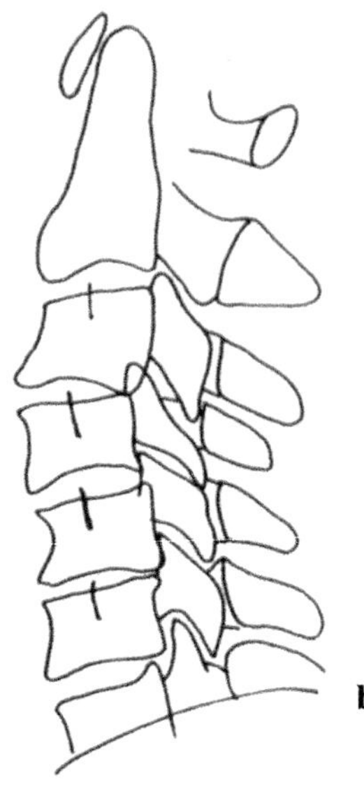

b

a

Here is a practical exercise: a review of the preceding features.

There is slight retrolisthesis of C5 at the level of degenerative changes at C5–C6 with an intact interapophyseal space and with no thickening of the soft tissues: a degenerative origin is most likely (**a, b**).

There is also slight retrolisthesis of C3 above degenerative changes at C3–C4 and with no thickening of the soft tissues: here again, a degenerative origin of the displacement is most likely.

If you have not noticed anything else, return to the beginning because you have missed one essential thing: there is severe spinal stenosis: the posterior aspect of the articular processes projects almost onto the spinolaminar line, and there is almost a complete absence of the safety space.

40

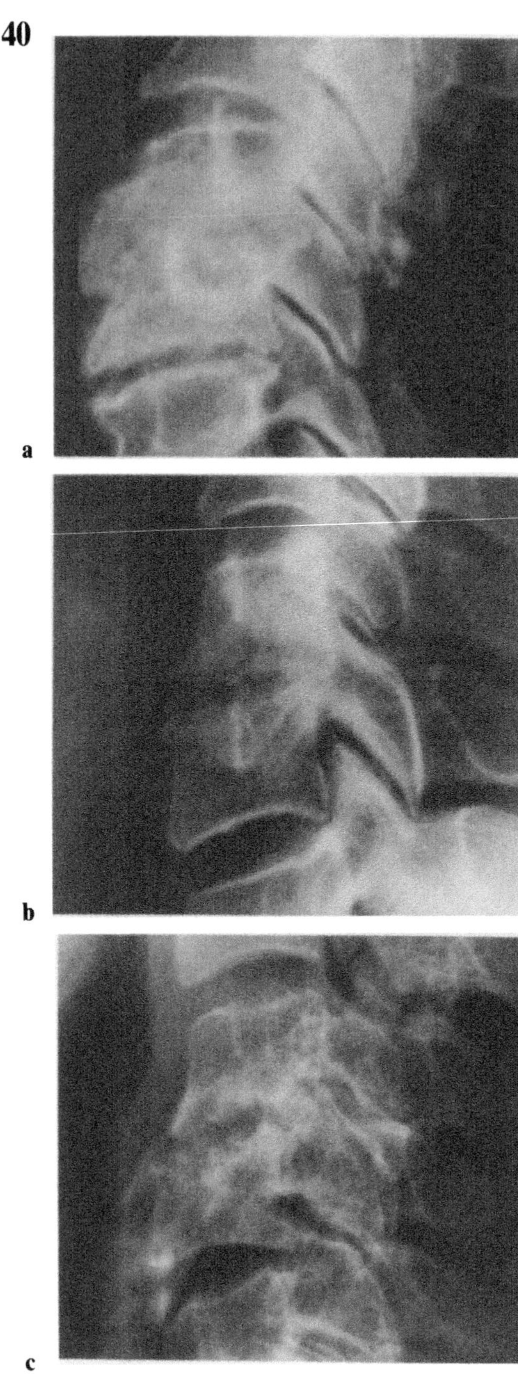

Not all cases of retrolisthesis are of degenerative or traumatic origin. The proof: among the three examples presented, only one is of degenerative origin. What is the aetiology of the other two?

---

a There is a huge osteophytosis anteriorly and laterally in association with disc shrinkage: this is degenerative retrolisthesis.

b Retrolisthesis is associated with discal narrowing which is more pronounced posteriorly, with demineralisation and erosion of the vertebral end-plates. This is a case of spondylodiskitis.

Thickening of the prevertebral soft tissues is difficult to verify in this case.

c The features are similar to the previous example, but here the soft tissues are not thickened. The osseous structure could suggest a diagnosis of spondyloarthropathy due to chronic haemodialysis. However this lesion resembles a spondylodiskitis, but, in general, there is no associated osteophytosis. The biological evaluation eliminates an inflammatory origin. Discal biopsy would demonstrate deposits of hydroxyapatite within the disc.

41

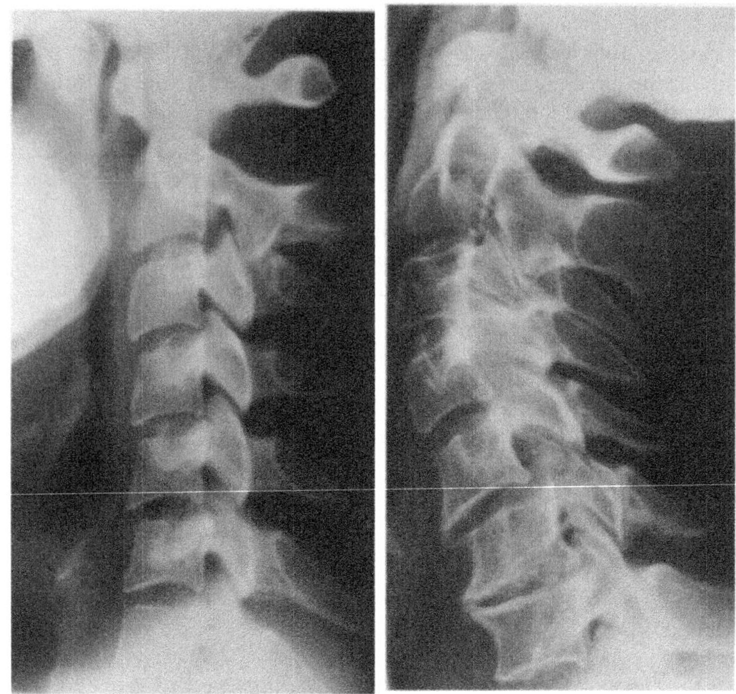

Case 41

These two post-trauma patients have exactly the same lesion. What is it?

In the two cases presented here, there is slight but clear spondylolisthesis of C5. The diagnosis of spondylolisthesis is easier in a young female (**a**) than in an elderly one (**b**), where degenerative spondylolisthesis may be suspected. However, such a vertebral displacement should the systematic search for a fracture of the articular process imperative. If the fracture line is not visible, an excellent sign of fracture of the superior articular process is an exaggerated radiolucency of the superior articular processes, as in these two cases, as the right and left superior articular processes are then no longer superimposed. In this case, note the radiolucency of the articular processes of C5 with respect to the articular processes above and below. The CT scans (**c** and **d**) confirmed the fracture of the articular processes.

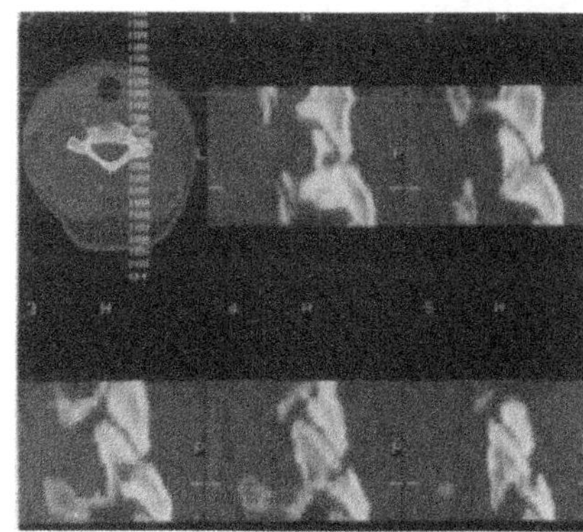

c

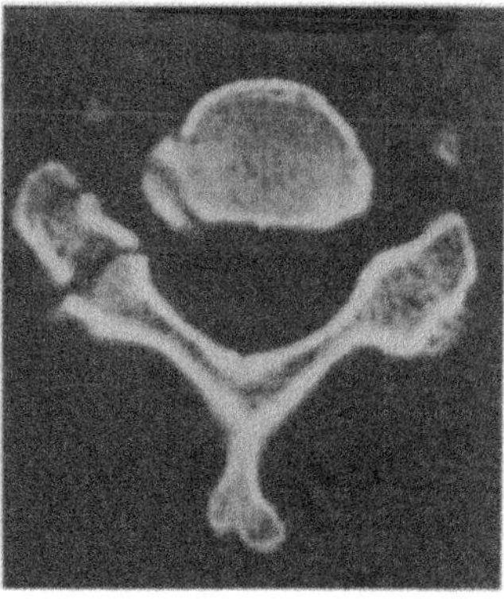

d

42

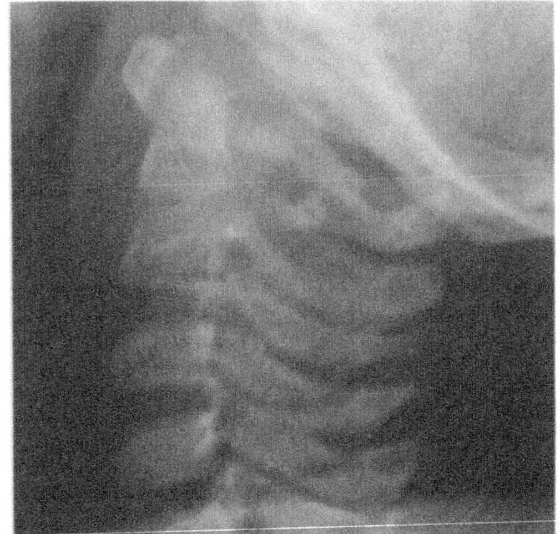

a

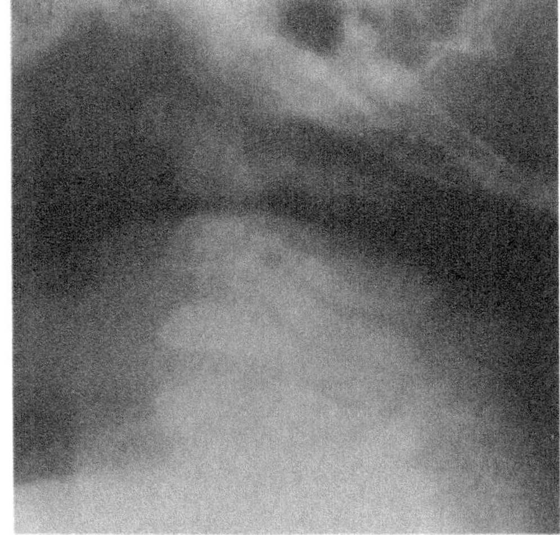

b

What has happened to these two neonates (**a, b**) who were radiographed after a trauma?

In these two cases, there is an image of a normal disc remnant between the odontoid process and the body of C2. However, the posterior arch of C3 seems to have lost its body, and it would be possible to suspect C3 vertebra plana. In fact, these two neonates have a completely normal cervical spine. Because of the lateroflexion of the head while taking the radiographs, the cervical spine has a marked curvature in the frontal plane. The body of C3 is located at the top of this curvature and is hidden by the body of C2 onto which it is projected (**c**).

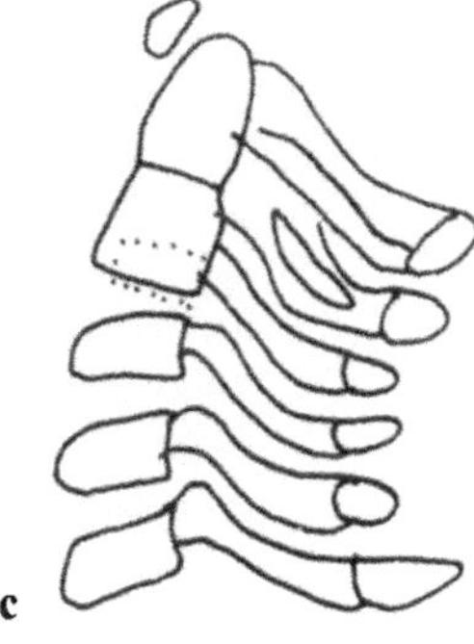

c

43

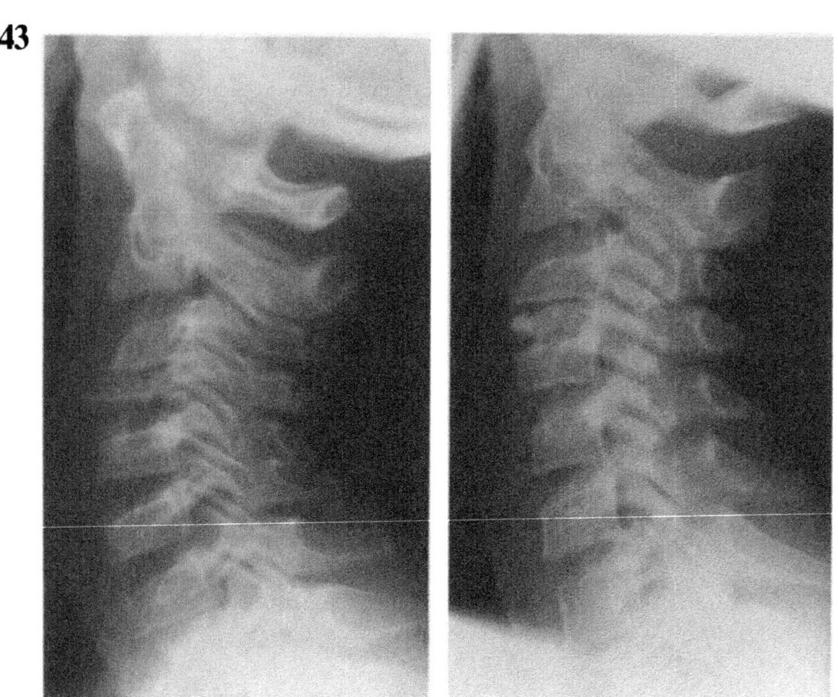

These two children had fallen, but not seriously. A few days later, they complained of a kind of torticollis. Is this false vertebra plana or true compressed vertebral bodies?

The false images of compressed vertebrae (case 42) are observed almost exclusively at C3 in neonates. These two radiographs do not resemble those of neonates; most of the vertebral bodies have lost their cuneiform shape and resemble the adult shape. The ossification centres of the epiphyseal rings have not yet appeared, so we can put the children's age at between 8 and 10 years.

Let us count the posterior arches and their corresponding vertebral bodies. **a** The spinous process of C4 is attached to a vertebral body which is flattened and slightly enlarged anteroposteriorly (**c**). This is a case of eosinophilic granuloma; this benign tumor has probably become symptomatic following a mild trauma.

b Either there is a spinous process missing; or there is a compressed vertebral body; or all the vertebrae are normal, but there is calcification at C3–C4! This is definitely a case of calcification of the nucleus pulposus (**d**), and there is no direct association with the recent trauma. Calcification of the nucleus pulposus may be encountered around the age of 7 after trauma, infection or during the course of some metabolic diseases. These calcifications may disappear in time.

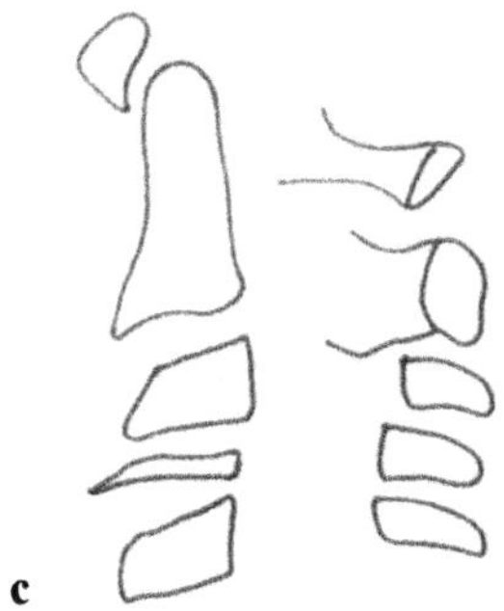

c

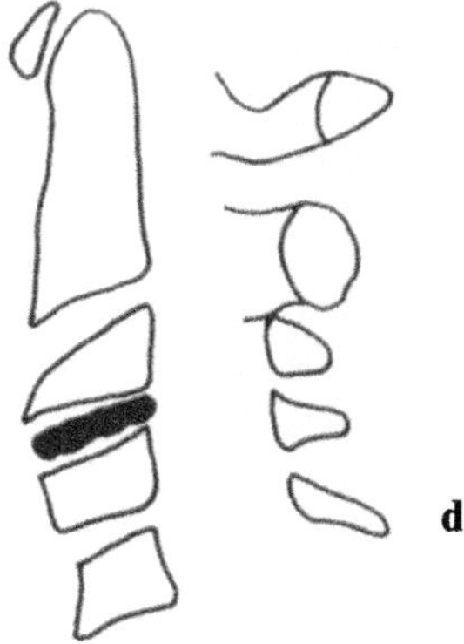

d

44

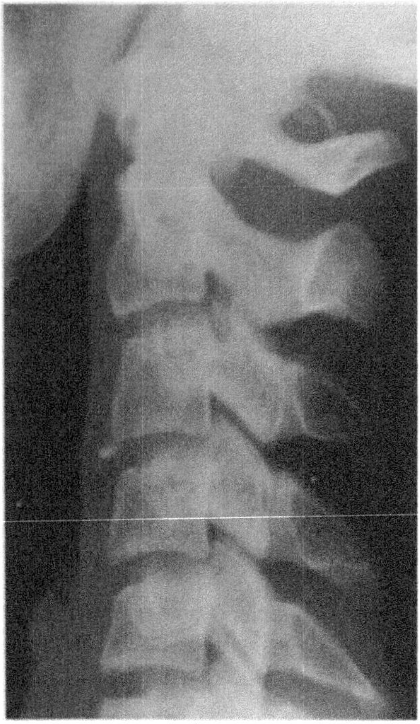

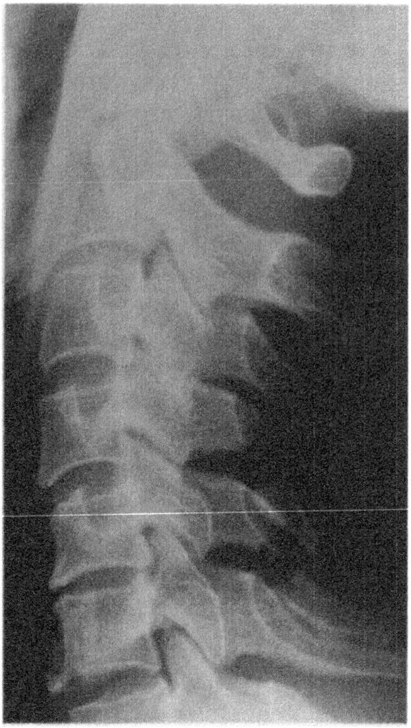

a

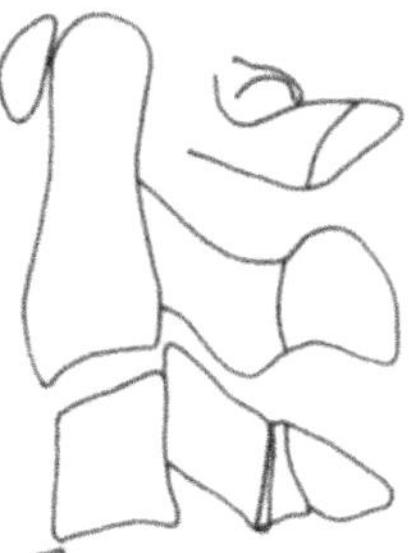

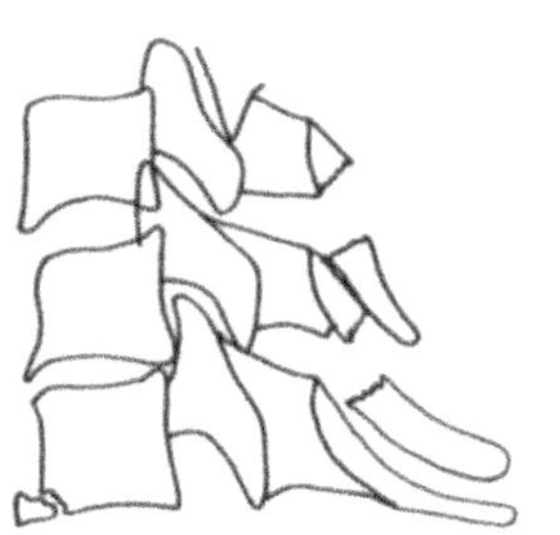

c

These two patients were the victims of a road traffic accident. Describe the lesions and their mechanism.

These lesions of the cervical spine are secondary to hyperextension. Moreover, both patients had severe facial injuries.

a The patient is 16 years old, and there is a detached epiphyseal ring at C3 (**c**).

b There is an avulsion fracture of the anteroinferior margin of C6. Note that the transverse diameter of the detached fragment is larger than its vertical height. There is also a fracture of the spinous processes of C4 and C5, with severe caudal displacement of the fractured fragments (**d**).

Fractures of the spinous processes are mostly seen after a hyperflexion injury, but may also be observed, as in this case, after a hyperextension injury.

Note also, that the ossification of the vertebral canal at the posterior arch of C1 often looks like an incomplete ring; this should not be mistaken for a fracture.

45

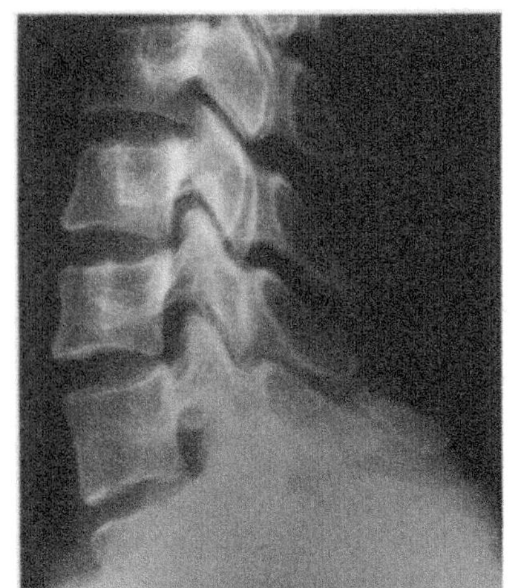

a

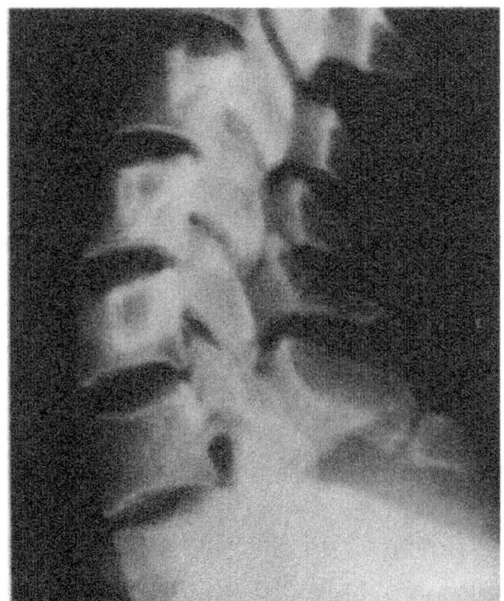

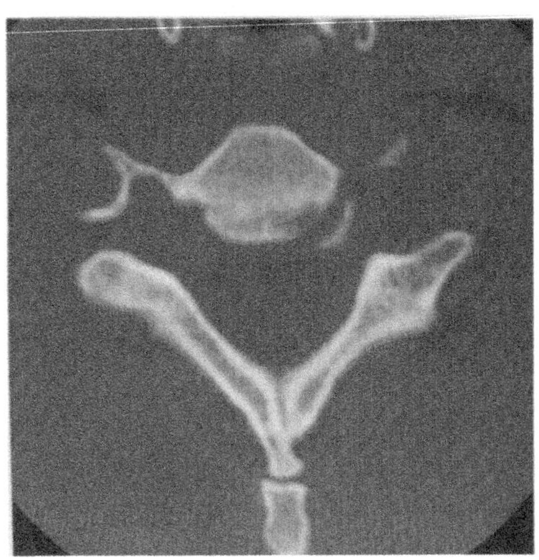

c

How can a fracture of the spinous process be distinguished from nonfusion?

Fractures of the spinous processes (**a**) are often multiple. If it is an avulsion fracture, as is generally the case, the direction of the fracture line is perpendicular to the orientation of the fibres of the interspinous ligament, as can be seen here at C7. The margins of the fracture are irregular.

Nonfusion of the extremity of the spinous process (**b**) is almost always single. The margins of the defect are regular (**c**). The distal fragment is not displaced and remains in contact with the posterior arch. Nonfusion of the spinous process is frequently encountered at C7 and C2.

46

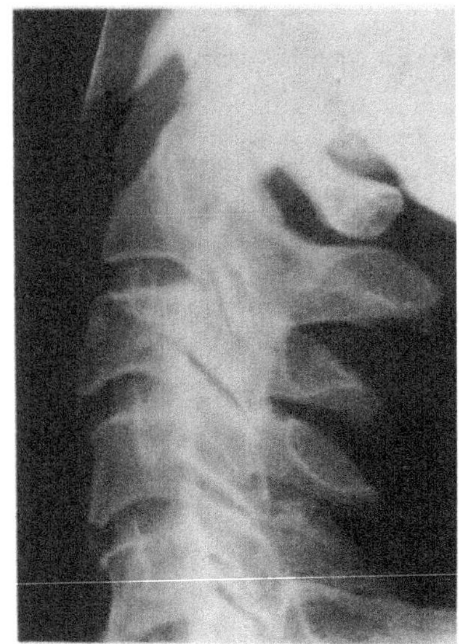

a

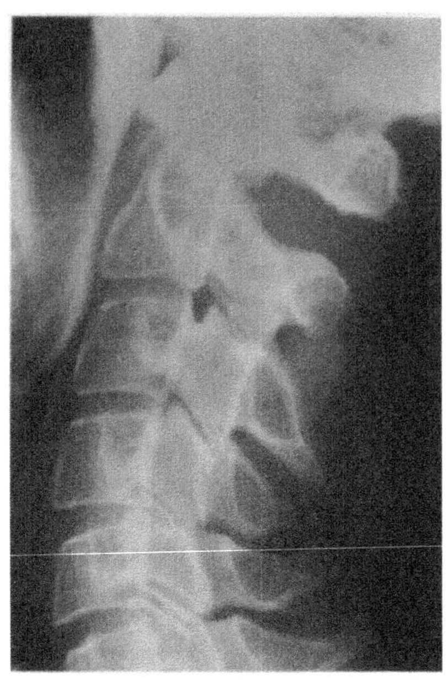

b

Case 46

These two patients have a minor congenital anomaly. What is it?

There is congenital nonfusion of the posterior arch of C5 (**a, c**): the spinolaminar line of C5 is missing, which signifies that the laminae are not fused at the midline. It is a minor malformation without clinical significance.

The other patient (**b, d**) presents a nonfusion of the C2 spinous process; this relatively frequent anomaly should be distinguished from a traumatic lesion.

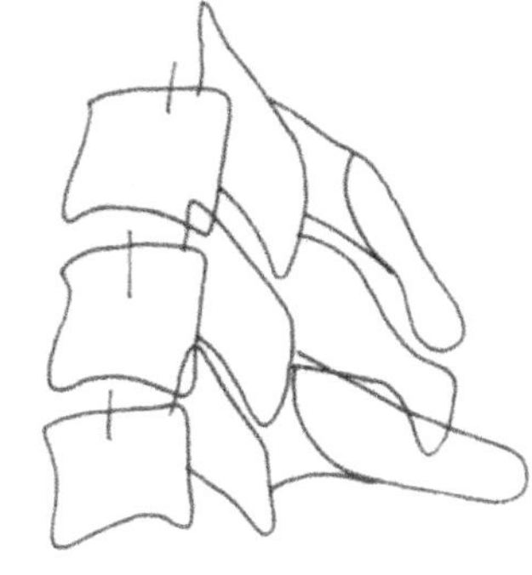

c

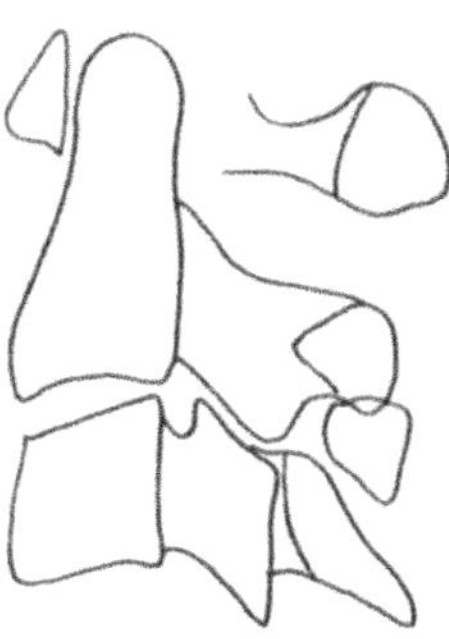

d

47

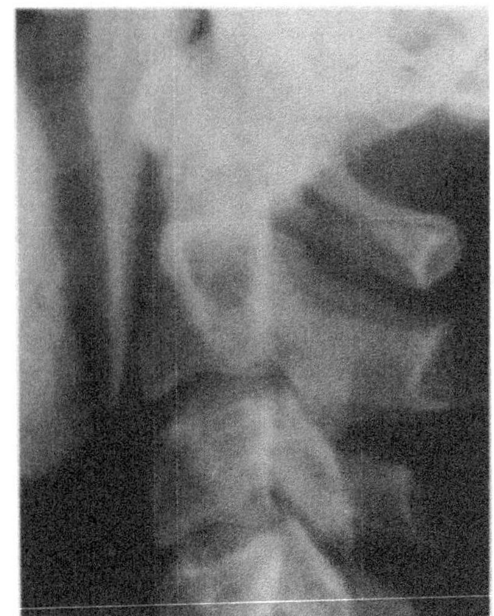

a

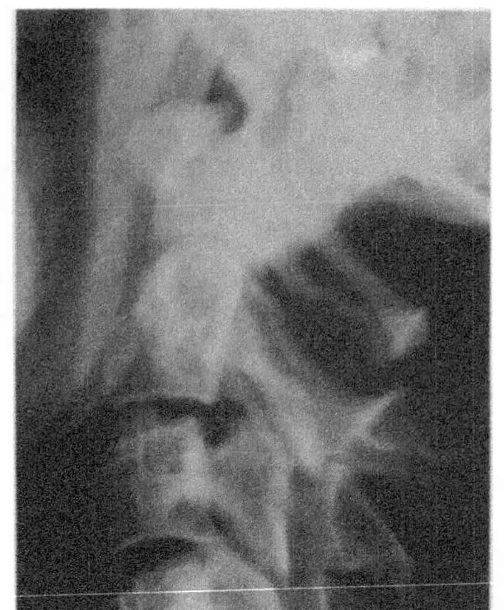

b

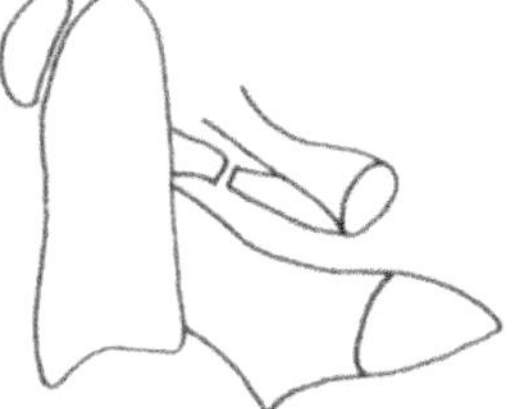

c

d

A fracture of the posterior arch of atlas was suspected in these two patients: What do you think?

These are not fractures (**a–c, b–d**) but two cases of congenital lateral defect of the posterior arch.

Note that in each case the posterior arch is tapered on either side of the defect.

Moreover, in **b**, the posterior arch is very thin: hypoplasia of the posterior arch is often compensated, as is the case here, by hypertrophy of the anterior arch.

48

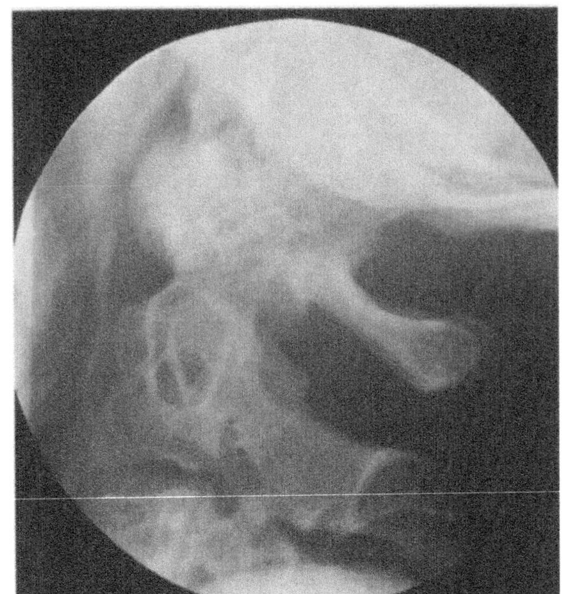

a

Can you recognise a congenital anomaly of the cervico-occipital junction?

This is a case of a split atlas, that is, the first vertebra is composed of two nonfused halves. There is median dehiscence of the anterior arch as well as of the posterior arch. The median dehiscence of the posterior arch can be easily seen as the spinolaminar line of C1 is missing (**a**). The median dehiscence of the C1 anterior arch is more difficult to identify, but the thick-set, rounded and mushroom-like appearance of the anterior arch of atlas is characteristic of this anomaly. The three-dimensional CT scan (**b**) confirms the existence of the two halves. The dehiscence of the posterior arch *(white arrows)* is seen through the foramen magnum; the anterior aspect of the odontoid process *(arrow head)* is visible through the defect of the anterior arch of atlas *(black arrows)*.

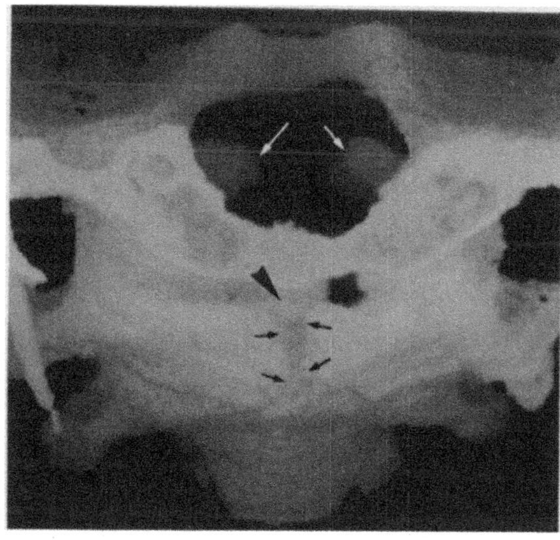

b

49

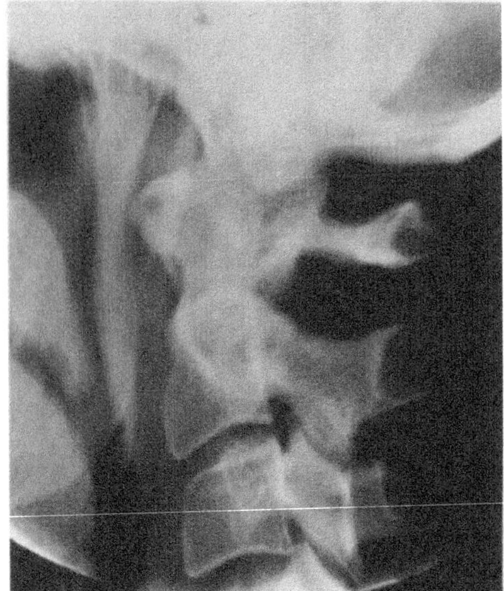

a

Cervical pain and dysphagia associated with fever.

The clinical context facilitates the diagnosis, but the radiological signs are also characteristic on the plain film (**a**), the tomogram (**b**) as well as on the CT scan (**c**): there is calcification below the anterior arch of atlas, within the longus colli muscle, causing the prevertebral soft tissues to bulge. This is a case of calcification of the ligament of the longus colli muscle. The longus colli is the principal flexor of the cervical spine; its insertion point is on the inferior surface of the anterior tubercle of atlas. This is a kind of acute tendinitis which is responsible for pain and muscular spasm, as frequently seen in the shoulder, hip or elbow. The calcified tendinitis of the longus colli is due to the deposition of hydroxyapatite crystals, which may disappear with anti-inflammatory treatment.

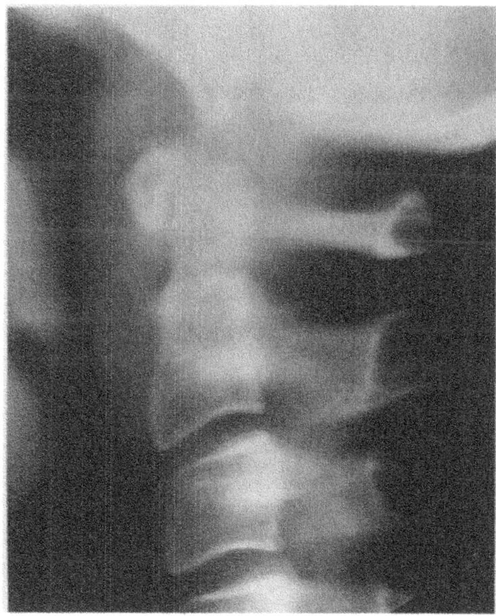

b

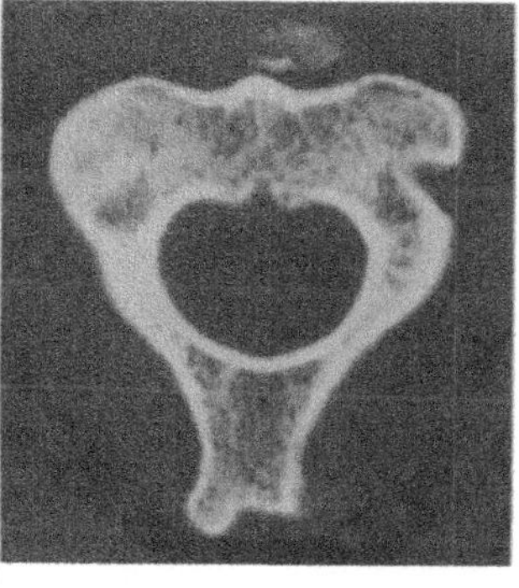

c

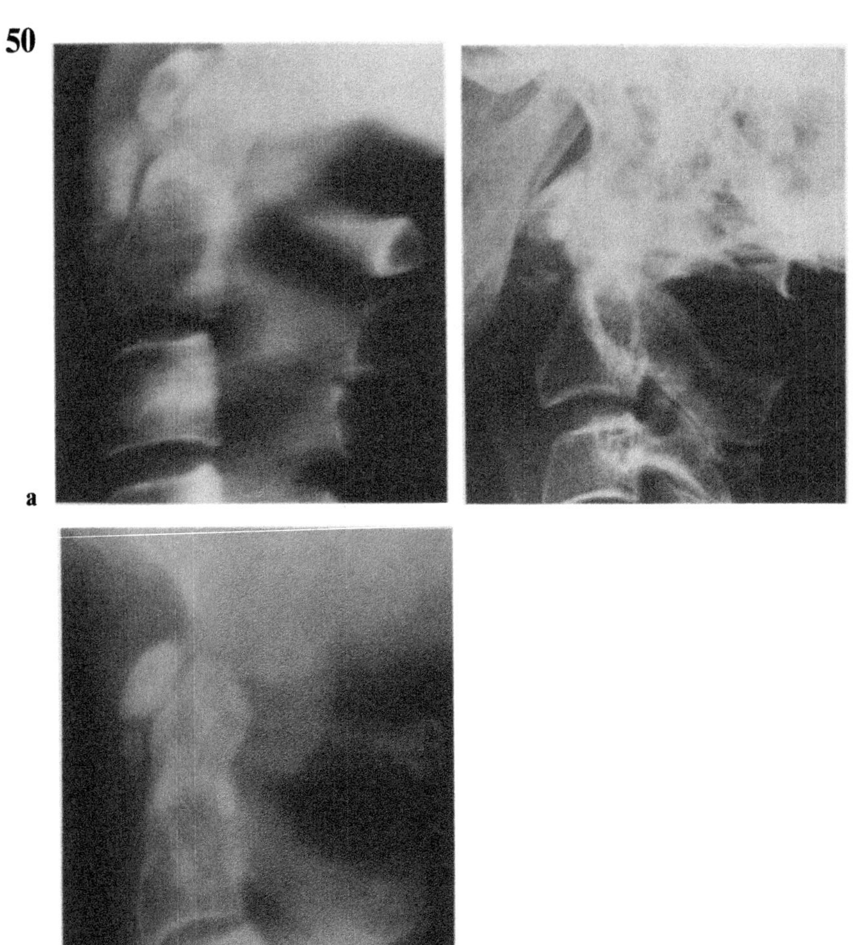
50
a
b
c

Among the three radiographs, only one corresponds to the deposit of hydroxyapatite in the longus colli muscle. Which one? What is the differential diagnosis?

The calcification of the longus colli muscle is shown in **a**. The anterior arch of atlas is intact. The prevertebral soft tissues bulge in front of C2. However, would you noticed that there is also a large osteolytic metastasis on the body of C2?

b The prevertebral soft tissues are much enlarged. This is a case of a horizontal fracture of the inferior part of the anterior arch of atlas. The margins of the fracture are very irregular. A horizontal fracture of the anterior arch of atlas is relatively rare; it is mostly the result of a hyperextension injury tearing the insertion of the longus colli at the level of the anterior arch of atlas. The fracture of the anterior arch of atlas is rarely isolated. Other lesions, such as fracture of the odontoid process or of the posterior arch of the atlas, are frequently associated, as is the case here (**d**).

c There is an accessory ossicle situated below the anterior arch of atlas, without modification of the prevertebral soft tissues. This accessory ossicle is a minor anatomical variant.

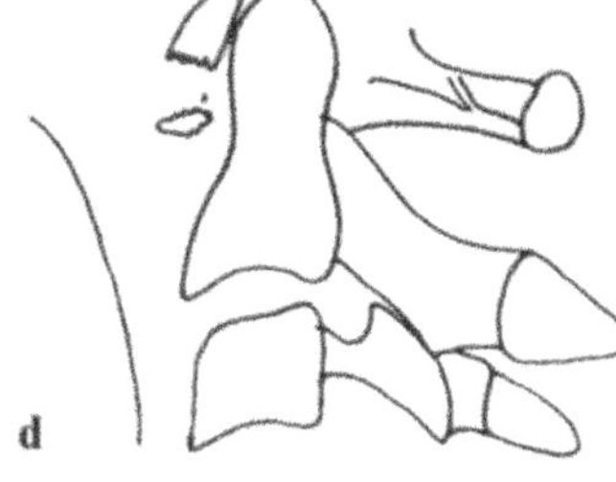

d

51

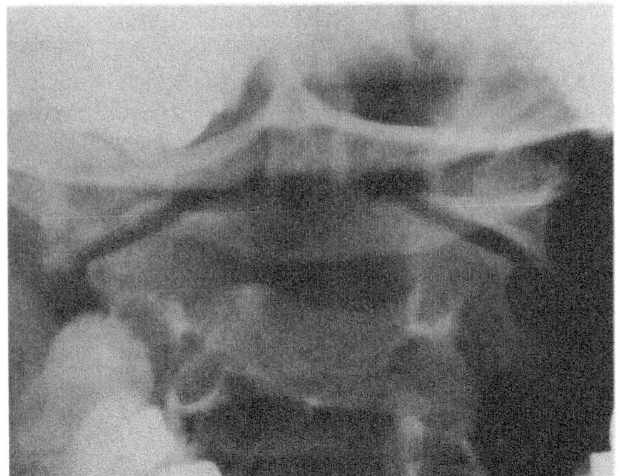

a

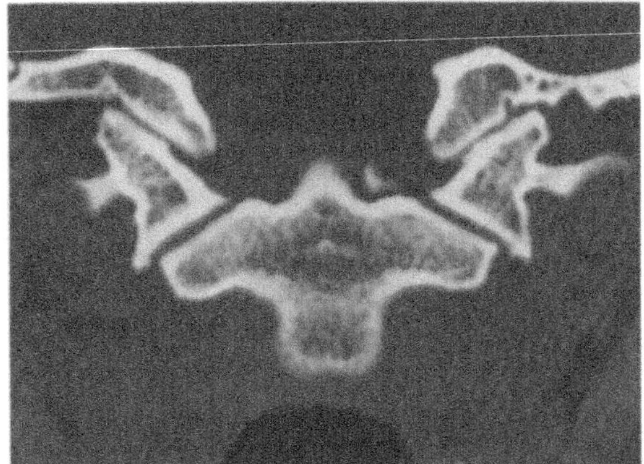

b

The open-mouth view (**a**) is often difficult to interpret. Here the diagnosis is obvious, facilitated by the corresponding coronal CT scan.

We have just seen a horizontal fracture of the anterior arch of atlas resulting from hyperextension of the head (case 50). In this case, the mechanism of the fracture is by axial compression exerted on the vertex: for example, when the top of the head hits a windscreen or in a diving accident, the atlas is crushed between the occipital condyles and the articular processes of C2, and the lateral masses of atlas tend to be displaced laterally (**b**). This fracture of the atlas is due to vertical fractures of the ring at its weak points, namely, at the point of fusion between the lateral masses and the anterior and posterior arches. Frequently, as is the case here (**c**), there is also an avulsion of the insertion of the transverse ligament at the median tubercle of the atlas, which is well seen in axial views. This fracture of the atlas, called Jefferson's fracture, is easy to recognise in the anteroposterior view because the lateral masses of the atlas are spread out and protrude on either side the articular processes of C2.

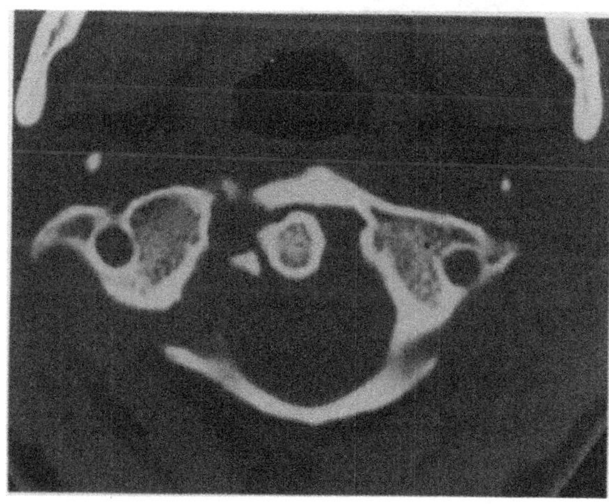

c

52

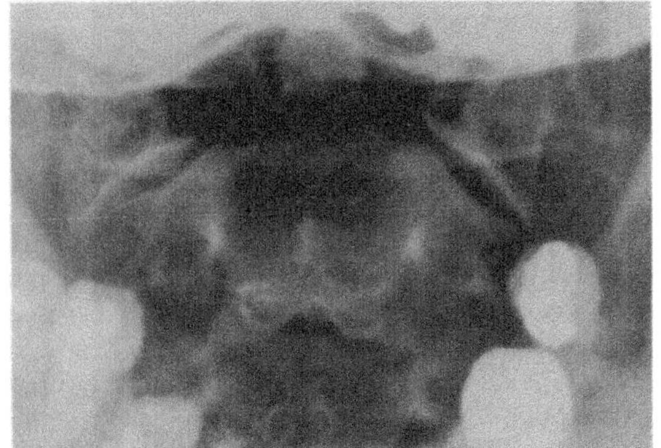

a

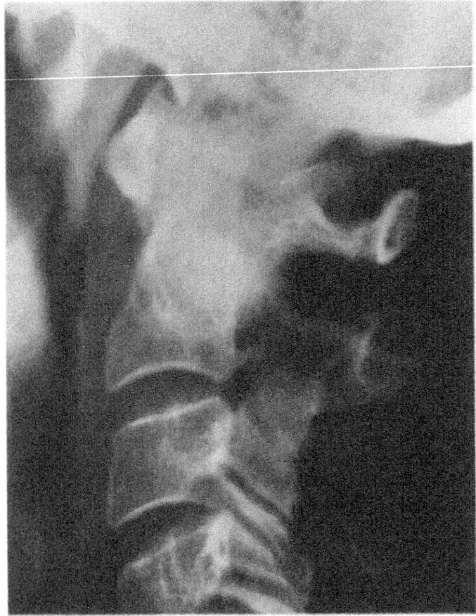

b

Obviously, this is a Jefferson's fracture. What is special here? What do you note about the lateral view?

In the anteroposterior view (**a**), there is lateral displacement of the lateral masses of atlas, which can be more clearly seen on the right. It is said that, if lateral step-off exceeds 7 mm, then there is a greater chance the tubercle of insertion of the transverse ligament has sheared. We can see such an avulsion on the right (**c**). In the lateral view (**b**), we are immediately struck by the almost normal image on the radiograph. In cases of Jefferson's fracture, the vertical fracture lines at the junction of the lateral masses and the anterior and posterior arches are hardly visualised in the lateral view. Here, however, one of the fractures of the posterior arch is visualised, a few millimetres in front of the spinolaminar line (**d**). The prevertebral soft tissues are obviously abnormal. Finally, note that the lateral and caudal displacement of the lateral masses of atlas projects them onto the body of C2 and the neighbouring pars interarticularis in the lateral view. This gives rise to an opaque area which is projected onto Harris's ring and the pars interarticularis in the lateral view (**d**).

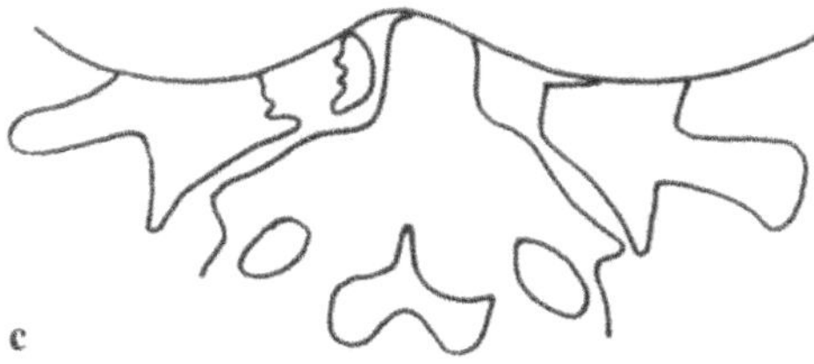

c

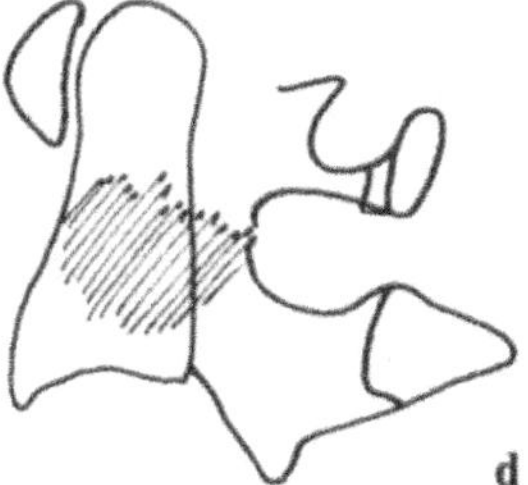

d

53

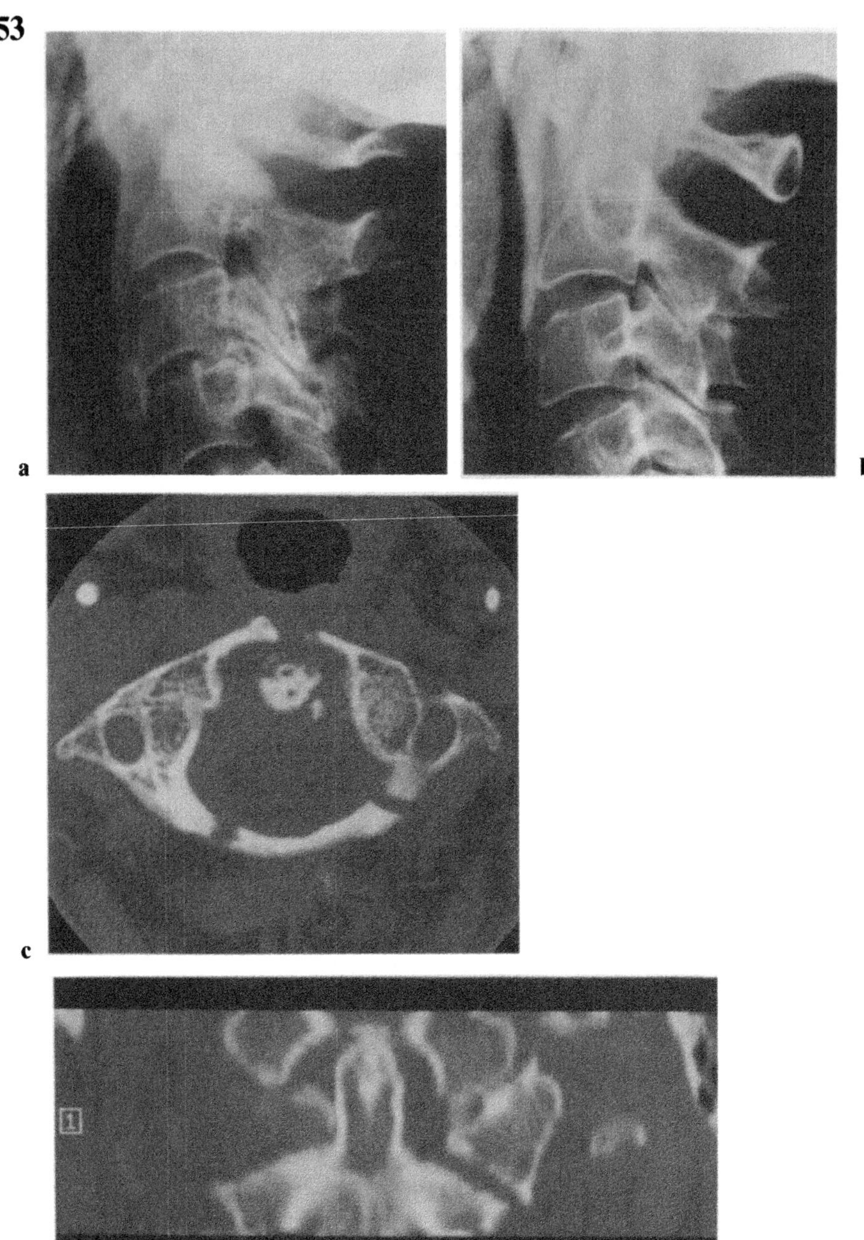

Case 53

In the two lateral radiographs, you have seen a diastasis at C1–C2 which is more pronounced in **a** than in **b**. These diastases with parallel interfaces are pathological and indicate a lesion of the transverse ligament. One of the two radiographs shows a Jefferson's fracture (**c**), and the other, a metastasis of the lateral mass of atlas (**d**). Which is the lateral radiograph corresponding to the Jefferson's fracture? Naturally, you are allowed only one answer!

The answer is **a–c**, **b–d**: the Jefferson's fracture here consists of three vertical lines with an avulsion of the insertion of the transverse ligament on the left. This fracture has resulted in a lateral and caudal displacement of the lateral masses of atlas, which you will have recognised by the opacity projected onto the body of C2 and the adjacent isthmic region (**e**).

On the other hand, the metastasis of the lateral mass of atlas is evident as a result of the radiolucency of its posterior part (**f**); Harris's ring is normal.

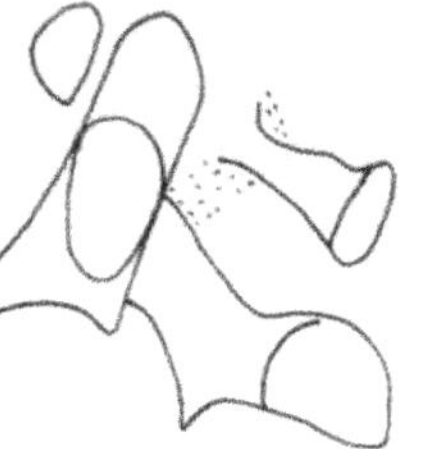

e **f**

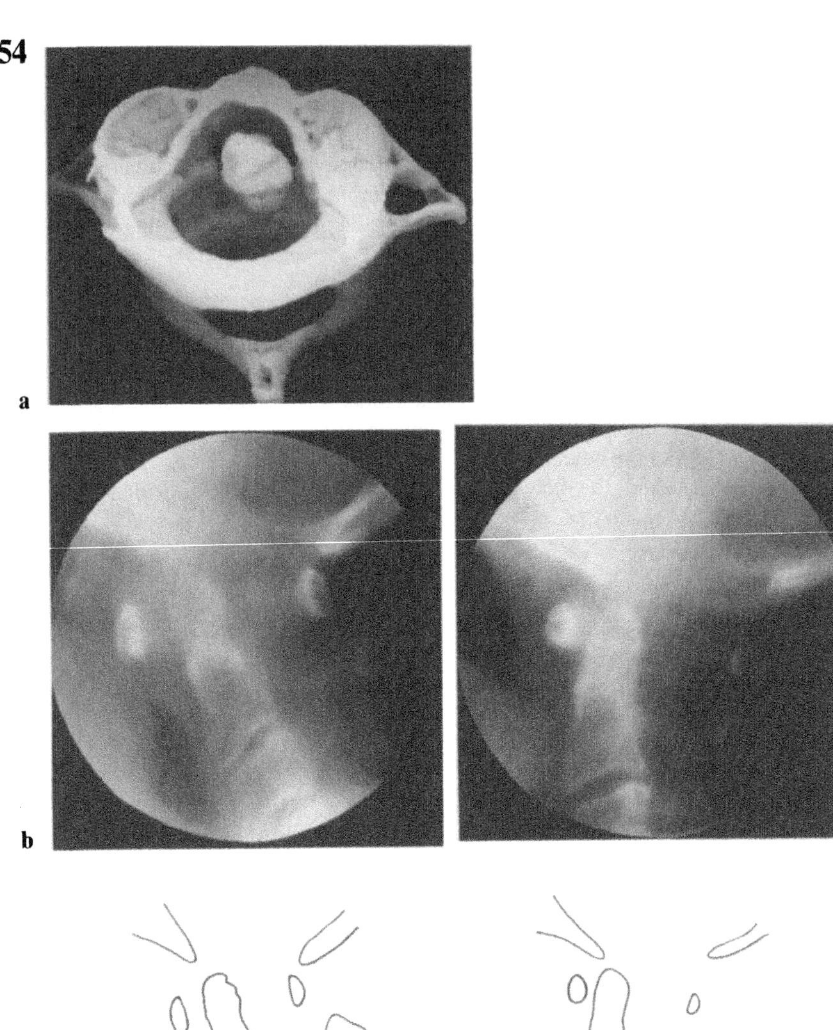
54
a
b
d

The C1–C2 dislocations (**a**) are due to a lesion of the transverse ligament. The diastasis may be considerable (**b**) or slight (**c**). In each case, the spinal canal is relatively large between the posterior aspect of the odontoid process and the spinolaminar line of C1. Radiographs obtained with flexion of the head would show whether there was an increase in the severity of the diastasis and whether the spinal cord was under threat. What are the most probable aetiologies of the C1–C2 dislocations shown in **b** and **c**?

---

b There is an involvement of the transverse ligament due to rheumatoid arthritis: the odontoid process is demineralised and shows cortical erosions (**d**).

c There is here no evidence of local demineralisation. The posterior surface of the anterior arch of atlas is convex posteriorly (**e**): this unusual morphology of the anterior arch of atlas testifies an abnormal congruence between the articular surfaces and may be observed in cases of insufficiency of the transverse ligament of atlas.

55

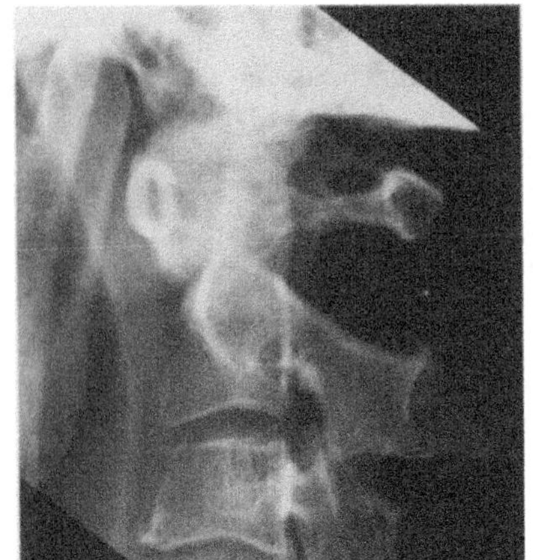

a

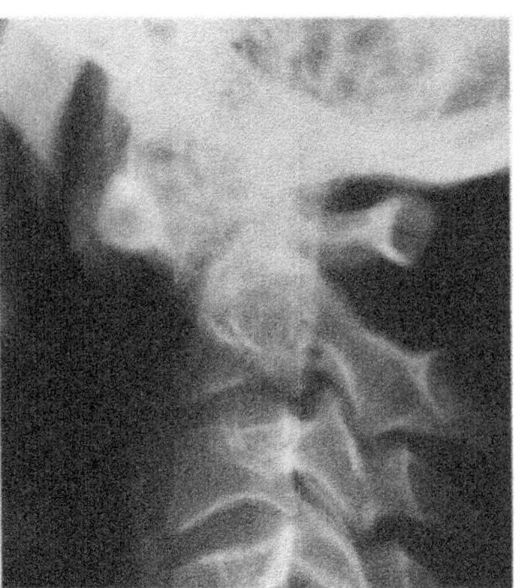

b

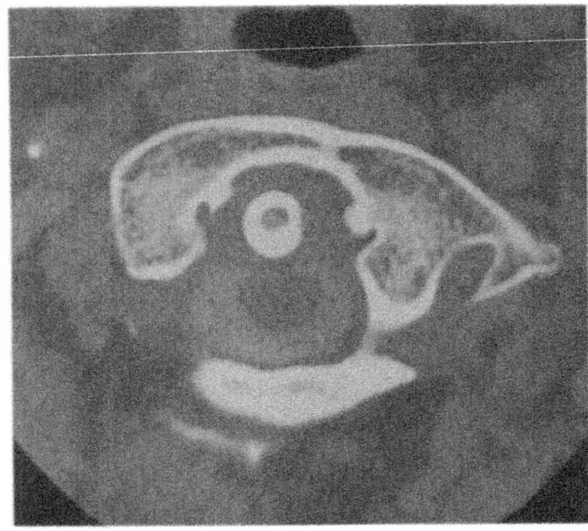

c

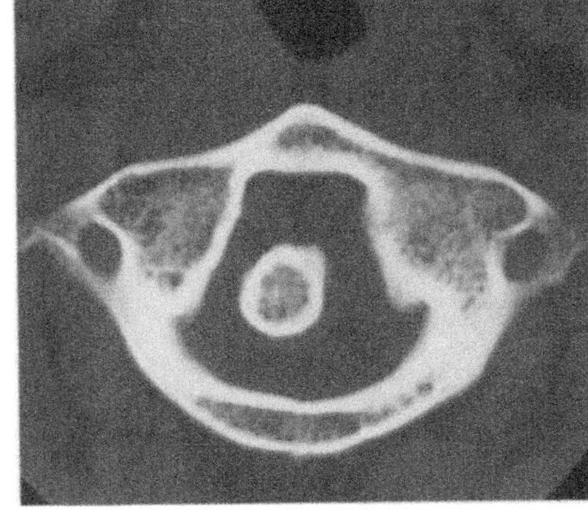

d

Here again, there are two C1–C2 dislocations with considerable diastasis between the anterior arch of atlas and the anterior surface of the odontoid process. You will have noted in **b** that the spinal canal is much narrower at C1 even without flexion of the head. Could you tell us what you think about the origin of these two diastases. The corresponding CT scans will help you (**a–c**; **b–d**).

There is no demineralisation or erosion of the posterior surface of the odontoid process in neither of the two cases: it is highly unlikely that there is a rheumatic lesion of the transverse ligament. In **a**, the dislocation was in fact discovered by chance; its origin is unknown and it is very likely to remain unknown.

b This lesion was also discovered by chance. You will have certainly noted the rounded appearance of the anterior arch of atlas, the posterior surface of which is convex posteriorly. The possibility of a congenital insufficiency of the transverse ligament seems to be confirmed by the CT scan which shows abnormal lateral masses of atlas, the inner surface of which is smooth: the absence of the median tubercle of atlas where the transverse ligament is normally attached reinforces the possibility of a congenital ligamentous insufficiency. Compare this with the normal appearance of lateral masses (**c**).

56

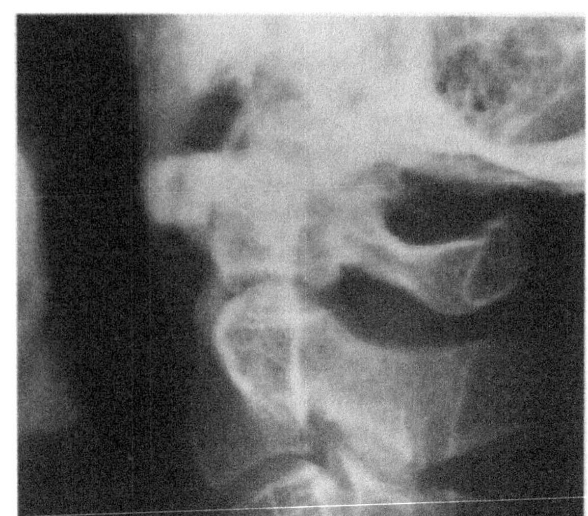

a

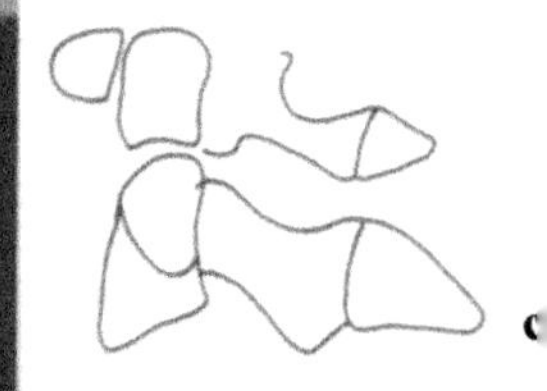

c

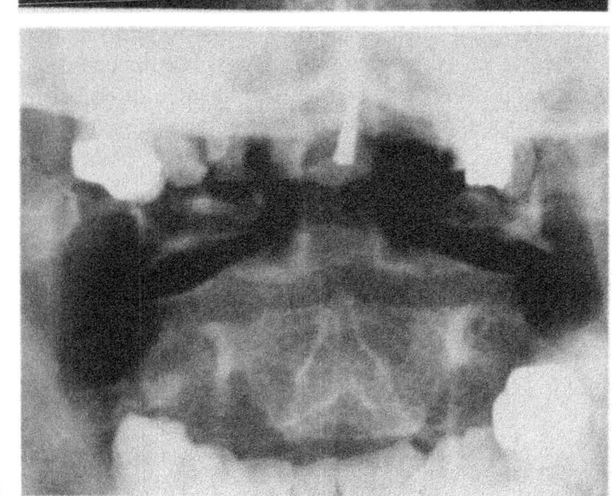

b

In the lateral view (**a**), you will have noted a radiolucent line at the base of the odontoid process (**b**). Is it a fracture? Or is it an os odontoideum?

We do not see any trace of a fracture in the anteroposterior open-mouth view (**b**), but we know that this does not exclude a fracture. On the other hand, the normal thickness of the prevertebral soft tissues means that a fracture is improbable.

The os odontoideum, that is, a nonfusion of the odontoid process with the body of C2, is always well seen in the anteroposterior view and can therefore be excluded here.

The diagnosis is given by the anteroposterior view: there is an unusual orientation of the joint space between the inferior surfaces of the lateral masses of C1 and the superior surfaces of the articular processes of C2. In the lateral view this space is almost horizontal and is therefore tangential to the X-ray beam. The radiolucent line cutting across the odontoid process in the lateral view corresponds to an unusual visualisation of the C1–C2 articular interspace. An identical image is often visible in the lateral view when the X-ray beam is oblique and directed superiorly and is thus tangential to the articular surfaces of C1 and C2.

In this case, compare the orientation of the C1–C2 space with the usual appearance (for example, case 51).

57

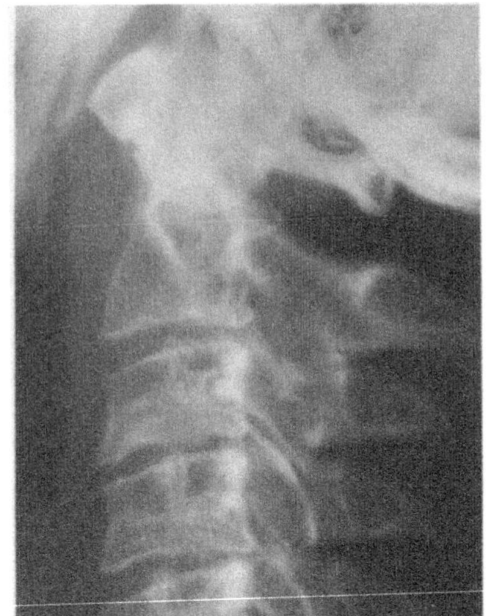

a

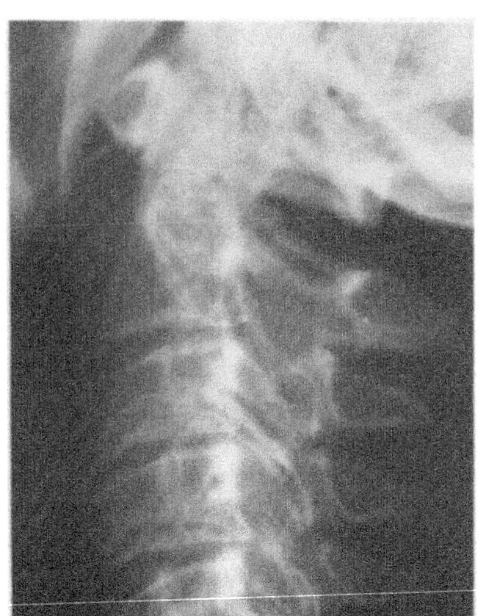

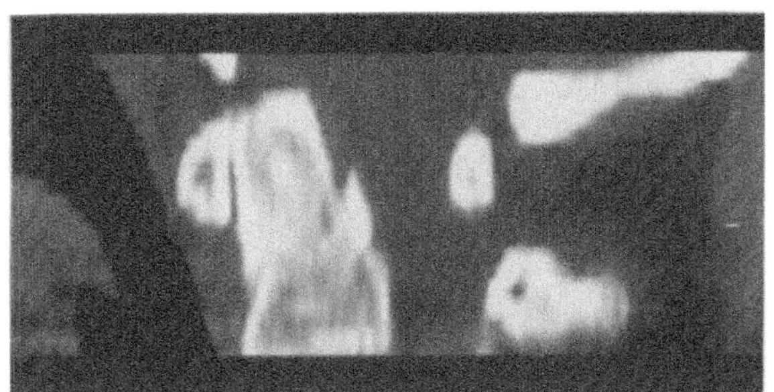

c

We shall soon have to finish. I should like to make sure that you have remembered something that is particularly important to me. What is the difference between these two radiographs of the same patient, taken 48 h apart?

The first radiograph (**a**) is practically normal. Two days later (**b**), the prevertebral soft tissues situated in front of C2 are definitely pathological: they are enlarged, and the posterior surface of the nasopharynx is concave posteriorly. There is a fracture of the odontoid process with secondary displacement of the fragments (**c**). It should be remembered that, in elderly and in osteoporotic patients, the enlargement of the prevertebral soft tissues secondary to a haematoma may be delayed by 48–72 h after the trauma.

58

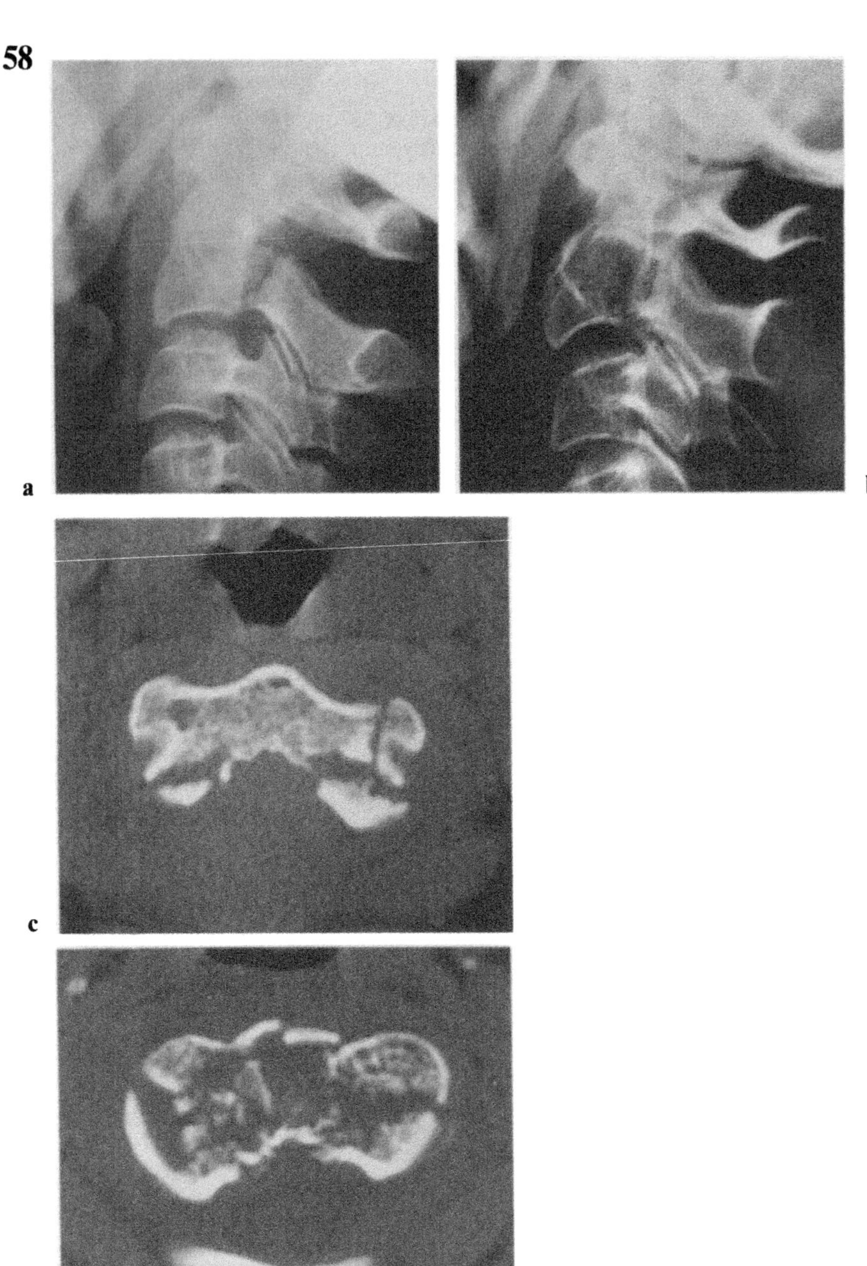

The diagnosis of fracture of the cervical spine can be decided on the basis of direct signs (visualisation of the fracture line) or indirect signs (enlargement of the prevertebral soft tissues, for example). Here, in **b**, there is another indirect sign. Look for and describe the lesions.

---

a The diagnosis of traumatic spondylolisthesis of the axis or "hangman's fracture", that is, a vertical fracture of the C2 pedicle, is easy here because the fracture line is perpendicular to the X-ray beam. Note that the prevertebral soft tissues are almost normal in this type of fracture of the posterior arch. The mechanism of this fracture of the pars interarticularis of C2 is traumatic hyperextension of the head, which may also produce a fracture of the posterior arch of C1, although not in this case. There are three types of traumatic spondylolisthesis of the axis:

Type I. There is no displacement or angulation of the fragments, and there is displacement of C2 over C3 by less than 3 mm.

Type II. There is displacement between C2 and C3 with angulation and very often, a rupture of the posterior longitudinal ligament and disc; frequently there is an associated fracture of the anterosuperior corner of C3.

Type III. There is dislocation of the articular processes with severe instability.

In type I, as in this case, there is generally no enlargement of the prevertebral soft tissues, and the diagnosis may be very difficult if the fracture line is not tangential to the X-ray beam. The CT scan (**c**) shows the main fracture line and other fracture lines which may extend to the vertebral canal.

b The prevertebral soft tissues are obviously much enlarged, but we cannot see the fracture line clearly. However, there is another indirect sign of a comminuted fracture of the body of C2, the "fat axis": the body of C2 appears to have ballooned, and its anteroposterior diameter mostly exceeds that of C3. The axial CT scan (**d**) shows this very well: the fracture lines of the body of C2 take very different directions, and the fragments are separated from one another, which enlarges the body of C2 all over. In general, the mechanism responsible for these oblique fractures of the body of C2, giving the impression of a fat C2, is one of rotation and lateral flexion.

59

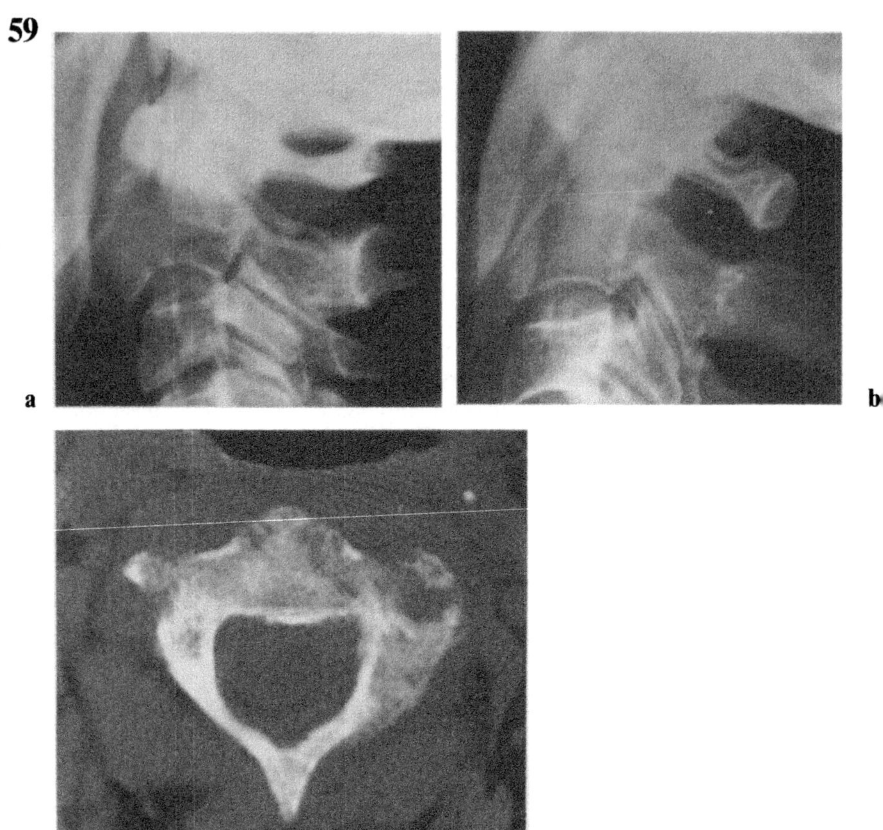

Is this another fat C2? What is the relationship between these two radiographs?

This is a case of an osteolytic metastasis of C2, sparing the odontoid process (**a**). Secondary to this the body of C2 is compressed and, as a result, is enlarged anteroposteriorly, displacing the prevertebral soft tissues. This metastatic localisation is frequent because of the rich vascularisation of the body of the axis. A discal remnant at the level of C1–C2 seems to protect the odontoid process from metastatic extension.

b This is also an osteolytic metastasis of the body of C2, sparing the odontoid process; it had been discovered before the fracture. The diffuse osteolysis of the body of C2 and of its posterior arch on the left can be well seen on the axial CT scan (**c**). Naturally, you will have noted in **b**, the bulging of the prevertebral soft tissues.

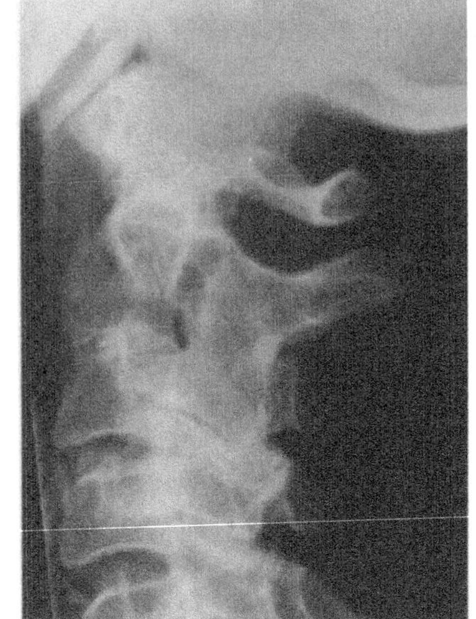

a

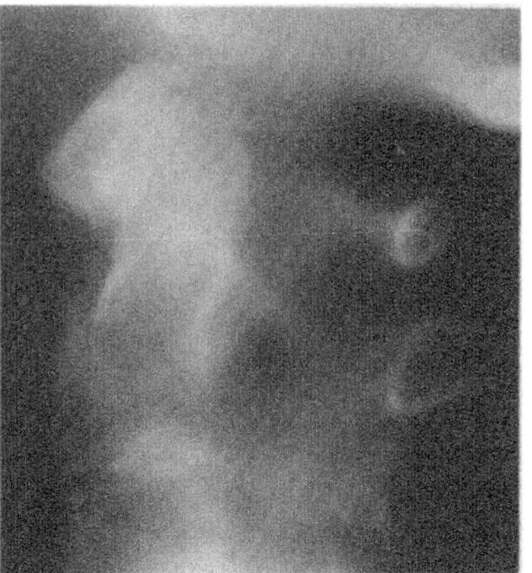

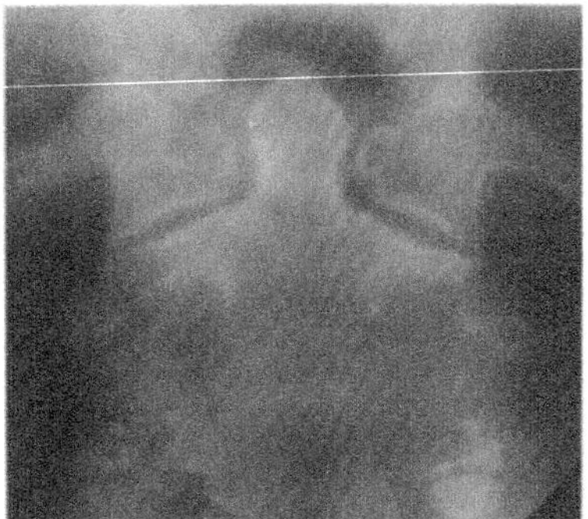

Is this a case of osteolytic metastatis of the body of C2, sparing the odontoid process? Not sure...

The body of C2 is more radiolucent than the vertebral bodies below (**a**). In the sagittal tomogram (**b**), it looks very much like an osteolytic lesion. You will have noted, however, that the prevertebral soft tissues are completely normal. It is the coronal tomogram (**c**) which offers the solution: on each side there are large imprints of dolichovertebral arteries beginning at the level of C3 and extending up to C2. These imprints are so deep that they considerably reduce the width of the body of C2, which explains the marked radiolucency of this vertebra in the lateral view. The axial CT scan (**d**) is more explicit, showing the dilatation of the vertebral canal of the left and right vertebral arteries which reduces the width of the body axis.

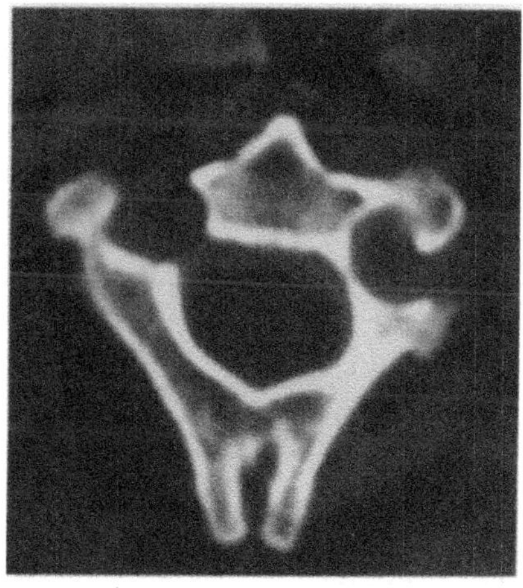

d

In spite of the revolution in medical imaging, plain radiographs of the cervical spine retain an important place in the diagnostic arsenal. The anatomical complexity, the superimpositions and the hidden traps make their interpretation difficult. May this little book make your evaluation of radiographs easier!

Subject Index

GPSR Compliance

The European Union's (EU) General Product Safety Regulation (GPSR) is a set of rules that requires consumer products to be safe and our obligations to ensure this.

If you have any concerns about our products, you can contact us on ProductSafety@springernature.com

In case Publisher is established outside the EU, the EU authorized representative is:

Springer Nature Customer Service Center GmbH
Europaplatz 3
69115 Heidelberg, Germany

Batch number: 09635031

Printed by Printforce, the Netherlands